To Improve Health and Health Care

Volume V

Stephen L. Isaacs and

James R. Knickman, Editors

Foreword by Steven A. Schroeder

To Improve Health and Health Care

Volume V

The Robert Wood Johnson Foundation Anthology

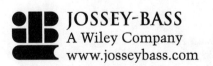

JOSSEY-BASS
A Wiley Company
www.josseybass.com

Published by

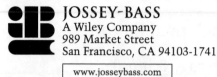

JOSSEY-BASS
A Wiley Company
989 Market Street
San Francisco, CA 94103-1741

www.josseybass.com

Jossey-Bass books and products are available through most bookstores. To contact
Jossey-Bass directly, call (888) 378-2537, fax to (800) 605-2665, or visit our website
at www.josseybass.com.

Substantial discounts on bulk quantities of Jossey-Bass books are available to
corporations, professional associations, and other organizations. For details and
discount information, contact the special sales department at Jossey-Bass.

We at Jossey-Bass strive to use the most environmentally sensitive paper stocks available
to us. Our publications are printed on acid-free recycled stock whenever possible, and
our paper always meets or exceeds minimum GPO and EPA requirements.

Library of Congress Cataloging-in-Publication Data

To improve health and health care. Volume V : The Robert Wood Johnson Foundation
anthology / Stephen L. Isaacs and James R. Knickman, editors ; foreword by Steven A. Schroeder.
   p. cm.
   Includes bibliographical references and index.
   ISBN 0-7879-5946-4
   1. Robert Wood Johnson Foundation. 2. Public health—Research grants—United States.
3. Public health—United States—Endowments. 4. Medicine—Research grants—United
States.   I. Isaacs, Stephen L.   II. Knickman, James.

RA440.87.U6 T626 2001
362.1'0973—dc21   2001050204

FIRST EDITION
PB Printing   10 9 8 7 6 5 4 3 2 1

—∿— Table of Contents

~~~ Foreword

This marks the fifth volume of *To Improve Health and Health Care: The Robert Wood Johnson Foundation Anthology.* The *Anthology* series tries to present clearly and forthrightly what the Foundation does, why it does it, and what it has learned from its experience. To do this, we ask outside journalists, program evaluators, and other experts to examine their topics with a critical eye, and to report their observations in language that is easily accessible to the lay public. Where chapters explore the inner workings of the Foundation, we ask Foundation staff members to be analytical and hard-headed as they write.

What unifies the *Anthology* series is the focus: every chapter relates to the Foundation's work to improve the health and health care of the American people—its mission since it became a national philanthropy in 1972. Beyond that, the book is truly an anthology: a collection of articles about a range of topics by a variety of authors, each with a different style and an individual perspective. Volume V is no exception.

The first six chapters focus on programs that are still running or that ended in the recent past.

In the first chapter, Joseph Alper, a writer specializing in health and science, examines the work of David Olds, whose program has offered nursing care and advice to poor, first-time mothers. This "nurse home visitation" approach, which the Foundation has funded for more than 20 years, and offshoots from it using less well trained (and less costly) workers, is being widely studied and has been adopted in a number of states with the hope that it will improve the health and well-being of both mothers and their children.

In chapter 2, Carolyn Newbergh, a California-based journalist with expertise in health care and policy, analyzes Old Disease, New Challenge, a program funded in the early 1990s, at a time when fear of a tuberculosis epidemic was mounting. It tested models of treating tuberculosis in hard-to-reach populations, including migrant workers in Florida, poor inner city people in New York, and migrants crossing the border between Tijuana and San Diego. Newbergh offers detailed case studies of three sites and provides insights gained from the program.

Chapter 3, by Paul Brodeur, a writer and specialist in health and environmental issues, looks at two programs to improve the health of Native Americans. Both programs gave the tribes and tribal organizations great flexibility in designing programs that would be in keeping with their culture and traditions. In his examination of the programs, Brodeur raises fundamental issues about the development of programs when recipients and donors do not share the same traditions, culture, and values.

In chapter 4, Susan Dentzer, the health correspondent for public television's *The NewsHour*, discusses two initiatives in which individuals who provide volunteer services for people with chronic illnesses receive credits that can be used when they themselves need help. She explores the genesis of the "service credit banking" idea, how the programs were carried out, and the reasons they did not work as planned.

The fifth chapter takes a look at a different approach to services for individuals with chronic illnesses: giving them the power to choose the services they use and the people who will provide them. A.E. (Ted) Benjamin, chair of the Department of Social Welfare, School of Public Policy and Social Research at the University of California, Los Angeles, and Rani Snyder, a research associate at the same institution, present three models that were tried at different locations throughout the country: one giving people with developmental disabilities the wherewithal to plan their own services; a second providing people wtih money to buy services; and a third testing a variety of approaches.

In the sixth chapter, Richard Frank, a free-lance writer and former editor of the *National Journal*, reviews one of the Foundation's longest-running programs—the Health Policy Fellowships Program. Begun in 1973 and most recently re-authorized in 2001, it gives health professionals the opportunity to spend a year working on Capitol Hill. Frank chronicles the nearly three decades of the program, pinpointing its shifting priorities and analyzing its successes and failures.

This volume of the *Anthology* introduces a new section called "A Closer Look." Unlike the first six chapters, which deal with the Foundation's large national programs, the chapters in this section look at smaller activities, such as those that occur at a single site. It offers a chance to examine activities at a community—or even an individual—level, rather than at the national level.

In chapter 7, Digby Diehl, a free-lance writer and frequent contributor to the *Anthology* series, scrutinizes Recovery High, an Albuquerque, New Mexico, high school for substance-abusing adolescents. It operated between 1992 and 1996, when lack of funds forced it to close. In his examination of this specific school and the people behind it, Diehl raises larger societal issues about the cost of treating drug-abusing children and who should bear it.

In 1989, the Foundation made a grant for the publication of a book, *On Doctoring*, to be edited by Richard Reynolds, then the Foundation's executive vice-president, and John Stone, a physician and writer. A collection of poems, stories, and articles about the practice of medicine, *On Doctoring* is given to every entering medical student in the nation. In chapter 8, Stone and Reynolds offer a personal reminiscence about how the idea of *On Doctoring* came about, the way in which they selected materials, and the value of a book designed to impart a sense of nobility, purpose, and pride in those who practice the profession.

The *Anthology* offers an opportunity to reflect upon the Foundation's past endeavors—to draw lessons from the past that can be useful in the present and the future. Previous volumes of the *Anthology* series have included chapters on the Foundation's efforts to develop emergency medical services, regional perinatal networks, dental services, and the fields of nurse practitioners and physician assistants.

In chapter 9, Ethan Bronner, the education editor of *The New York Times*, takes a look back at the Foundation's work to develop awareness of AIDS, and ways of preventing the spread of the disease. This was a major endeavor of the Foundation during the 1980s. Bronner traces the history of the Foundation's involvement, examines its large demonstration, research, and communications programs, and offers some lessons that were learned from the Foundation's experience in the AIDS crisis.

The final two chapters delve into the way the Foundation works. They attempt to demystify the Foundation—to give outsiders a better understanding of the way a large philanthropy operates.

Most foundation dollars are distributed as grants, but there is another, less well known mechanism available: loans, or, as they are more formally known, program-related investments. In chapter 10, Marco Navarro, a program officer at the Foundation, and Peter Goodwin, the treasurer and a vice-president of the Foundation, discuss when program-related investments are an appropriate funding mechanism, review the Foundation's experience with them, and examine the pros and cons of program-related investments.

The final chapter, written by Pamela Dickson, a senior program officer at the Foundation, examines how the Foundation maintains the legacy of its founder, Robert Wood Johnson, and how it relates to its neighbors in the New Brunswick area and throughout the state of New Jersey. She explores the tension between the Foundation's approach nationally—one relying on competitive responses to Calls for Proposals for programs with the potential to have a major impact—and its approach in New Jersey, which is, to a great extent, that of a community foundation.

In my foreword to the first volume of the *Anthology* series, I observed that any single volume would provide only a glimpse of the Foundation's diverse activities, and that a more complete picture would emerge over the succeeding years. In some areas, it is emerging. For example, the five volumes of the *Anthology* have featured 14 chapters about the Foundation's efforts to improve access to health care—a problem that has remained high on the Foundation's agenda since 1972.

Based on their analysis of these chapters, Stephen Isaacs and James Knickman, in the editors' introduction that follows, identify five complementary approaches that the Foundation has used to address this enduring problem. These approaches, they suggest, illustrate the strengths and limitations of philanthropy in bringing about social change.

Princeton, New Jersey   Steven A. Schroeder
August 2001   President and CEO
                                    The Robert Wood Johnson Foundation

—◠— Editors' Introduction

Strategies for Improving Access to Health Care: Observations from The Robert Wood Johnson Foundation *Anthology* Series

"The uneven availability of continuing medical care of acceptable quality is one of the most serious problems we face today. We need to better provide health services of the right kind, at the right time, to those who need it. Therefore, in its initial years, the Foundation will try to identify and encourage efforts to expand and improve the delivery of primary, frontline care." These words, written in 1972 by David Rogers, the first president of The Robert Wood Johnson Foundation, for the Foundation's first *Annual Report*, still resonate today.

Despite spending more than a trillion dollars on health care every year in the United States, more than 43 million Americans are still without health insurance, up from 31 million in 1987. Ten million children are uninsured. But the lack of health insurance is only part of this dismal picture. People who are poor, lower class, minority, or who live in inner cities or rural areas continue to have trouble getting medical services from a system that has become less, rather than more, responsive to their needs. Managed care may cut costs, but often at the expense of services and avoiding people with chronic diseases and other costly conditions.

Given the nearly intractable nature of the problem, the "initial years" Rogers referred to in the 1972 *Annual Report* have lasted three decades. Improving access to medical care not only remains a Foundation priority today but also is the one goal that has remained constant throughout the life of the Foundation. Reflecting this priority, access to care has commanded more space than any other topic in The Robert Wood Johnson Foundation *Anthology* series. Fourteen chapters on it have appeared in the five volumes of the *Anthology*. These chapters offer a perspective on how the nation's fifth-largest foundation has tried to improve access to care and, to a limited extent, what has resulted from its efforts. They reveal that, despite what appears at first glance to be a piecemeal way of doing business, the Foundation has taken five complementary approaches to addressing a problem that has commanded its attention for nearly 30 years.

The first approach: Fund research, particularly survey research, in order to gain a better understanding of the issue and its ramifications

Just a few years after its debut as a national philanthropic organization, the Foundation funded the first of four access-to-care surveys.[1] The findings from these surveys, conducted between 1976 and 1994, provided much of what was known about access, or lack of access, during that period. These surveys were followed, in 1995, by a large multi-year "health tracking" initiative designed to understand the changes in the health care system and their effects. For this initiative, the Foundation established the Center for Studying Health System Change, which conducts surveys in 60 communities every two years to find out, among other things, how managed care is affecting people's access to medical services.

This survey research has been supplemented by other quantitative research, much of which is conducted under the auspices of the Health Care Financing and Organization program, and, less frequently, by qualitative research such as that done by Susan Allen and Vincent Mor. Their study of the availability of services for chronically ill people living in Springfield, Massachusetts, concluded that the people most in need do not have access to even the most basic medical and social services.[2]

Over the years, the Foundation-funded research furnished "hard, reliable information on access to medical care."[3] It helped set the terms for debates about health policy and influenced the way that some policy makers and others thought about it. It is not clear, however, whether research has had an impact on policy, which may be driven more by ideology than by objective information.[4]

The second approach: Train and nurture leaders who can become "leaders in their home institutions, professional societies, and state and federal government."[5]

The Foundation has done this through a series of fellowship programs, directed mainly toward physicians. Two of them—The Health

Policy Fellowships Program and the Clinical Scholars Program—have been in operation for nearly three decades. The Health Policy Fellowships Program sends six mid-career health professionals to Washington, D.C., to work for a senator, a representative, or a congressional committee. Its original goals, dating to 1973, were nothing short of preparing doctors for senior policy making positions in government and changing the face of academic medical institutions.[6] The Clinical Scholars Program, considered by many to be the Foundation's flagship program, trains physicians in the social sciences and other fields outside their areas of clinical expertise in order to give them the breadth of knowledge they will need as they assume leadership roles.[7] Nearly 900 physicians have graduated from the program.

A more direct approach trained leaders of health professions whose members provide care to underserved people. Generalist medicine was one target. To develop a nucleus of leaders in general medicine (and to increase the credibility of generalist medicine in academic medical centers), the Foundation funded, in the 1970s, a series of primary care fellowship programs and residencies for general internists and general pediatricians. In 1991, it launched the Generalist Physician Initiative and two related programs intended to increase the attractiveness of primary care as a career choice for young physicians.[8] Nurse practitioners, thought to be a potential source of care for people living in rural areas and inner cities, were another target. To develop this field, the Foundation funded, between 1977 and 1991, the Nurse Faculty Fellows program and the Clinical Nurse Scholars Program. The nurses trained under these programs became the leaders who gave credibility to the relatively new field of advanced practice nursing.[9] Minority physicians, too, have been a target group. Since the 1980s, the Minority Medical Faculty Development Program has offered postdoctoral research fellowships to minority faculty members in non-minority medical schools and summer enrichment programs for minority college students interested in medical careers.[10]

Although these programs, with results that are not seen for many years, are expensive, often invisible to trustees and staff, and difficult to evaluate, they are considered to be a productive long-term investment. Writing in the 1998–1999 *Anthology*, Lewis Sandy and Richard Reynolds concluded that supporting promising young people through fellowship programs "may be a more effective institutional change strategy than direct institutional grants."[11]

The third approach: Support and assist organizations with the potential to improve access to care.

These organizations might be professional societies. For example, the Foundation funded the creation and early activities of societies of nurse-practitioners and generalist internists. Or they might be research, teaching, and practice institutions, such as academic medical centers, which were considered the key to reversing the stampede of medical students into sub-specialties. Or service delivery organizations. The Foundation's early support of health maintenance organizations, dating back to a grant to the Harvard Community Health Plan in the early 1970s, was aimed at meeting "the nation's need to assure access, control costs, and improve quality."[12]

In some cases, the Foundation has supported government organizations. The State Initiatives in Health Care Reform, begun in 1991, aided states that were exploring options for health reform. The states used the funds to convene commissions and hold conferences, to hire experts, to carry out research, and to hire staff. On a federal level, during the debate over health reform in the 1990s, both current and past Health Policy Fellows were called upon to assist senators and representatives, and to serve on health reform commissions.

The concept behind supporting government organizations is to help bring about policy change, albeit indirectly. This also has a potential down side. As Beth Stevens and Larry Brown noted in the 1997 *Anthology*, effective policy change requires a knowledge of, and perhaps an involvement in, the messy business of partisan politics—something foundations have not generally shown an aptitude for.[13] And foundations that do get involved in governmental policy matters—even if they are attempting only to improve the policy-making process—open themselves up to charges of political partisanship. Such accusations have been leveled against The Robert Wood Johnson Foundation at both the state and federal levels.[14]

The fourth approach: Get the word out.[15]

The Foundation uses communications as a tool to further its strategic interests. It has employed its resources to build public awareness of the astonishing numbers of the uninsured, the oft-tragic consequences of being uninsured, and potential solutions to the problem.

For example, the Foundation supported health coverage by National Public Radio and community radio stations for many years, funded PBS television specials such as *How Good Is Our Health Care?*, and, in keeping with its philosophy that grantees should do the talking, has arranged for training on how to deal with the media.[16] Linking research and communications, the Foundation organized a series of workshops for print journalists in cities where the Foundation-funded program Health Tracking was conducting surveys.[17]

To focus attention on the problem of the uninsured, the Foundation organized, in 1999, a conference of over 400 journalists, policy makers and analysts, and representatives of health-sector organizations. Known as the "strange bedfellows" conference because of the diversity of its participants, it was organized by Families USA and the Health Insurance Association of America.[18] Although these two organizations agree on very little, they were able to agree on a plan to cover the uninsured.

Taking a more direct tack, in 2000 the Foundation awarded a large grant to a Washington, D.C.-based public relations firm for radio and television ads to let people know that their children might be eligible for Medicaid or state health insurance. It is part of a larger program, called Covering Kids, to enroll children in Medicaid or state health insurance programs.

The fifth approach: Test innovative ideas and programs.

Such testing is traditionally done through demonstration programs—large applied research projects where different approaches to a problem are tried in different parts of the country. The hope is that successful approaches will be picked up by the government. The Foundation's very first national demonstration program was designed to improve access to emergency care. Taking place in the 1970s just as interest was on the rise—the television series *Emergency!* was a big hit at the time—the program demonstrated that the 911 emergency telephone service and regional emergency medical services could work. It was later absorbed by the federal government.[19]

A large number of demonstration programs have focused on children, many of them designed to improve the access of children to health care services or insurance.[20] These include programs to establish regional hospital networks for women with high-risk pregnancies,[21] to provide home nursing for poor pregnant women,[22] to establish school-based health clinics,[23] and to provide health insurance to children through their schools.[24] Other demonstrations to improve access to care have targeted AIDS[25] and tuberculosis,[26] homeless people,[27] and uninsured people.[28] In some cases, the federal government adopted the Foundation's approach and expanded it nationwide. This happened, for example, in the case of community-based programs for the prevention of AIDS and health care services for homeless people.

As the federal government has reduced its role in funding social programs, the Foundation's approach has evolved. In some cases, it now funds large national programs that, as Sharon Begley and Ruby Hearn observed in their chapter in the 2001 *Anthology*, engage the community and are large enough to have an impact on their own—irrespective of whether a program offers a replicable model.[29] The Urban Health Initiative, for example, attempts to improve children's health in entire cities, not just blocks or areas. Faith in Action, The Robert Wood Johnson Foundation's single largest program, provides funds that enable volunteers to help needy people in their communities. While not developed principally to increase access to medical care, the program often does so by funding volunteers to drive chronically ill senior citizens to medical appointments.

The Foundation's efforts to improve access to care illustrate the strengths and limitations of philanthropy in bringing about social change. Over the years, its fellowship programs have trained a cadre of leaders, its research has illuminated the field, its communications have kept the issue alive, and its demonstration programs have provided replicable models. Its efforts to affect policy have sometimes floundered in the messiness of partisan politics; it has not found a wholly satisfactory way to test new ideas now that government is less likely to pick up successful models, and it has been more comfortable with physicians and academics than it has been with activists and community-based organizers.

While some have questioned whether The Robert Wood Johnson Foundation should continue placing such a high priority on the exceedingly difficult problem of access to care, the Foundation's commitment is likely to continue. A retreat by the Foundation, whose efforts have been so visible, would send an unfortunate signal to the field. More important, lack of access to care remains a fundamental problem for our society. A large foundation whose very mission is improving health and health care has an obligation to play a leadership role in addressing this critical issue. And the willingness of the nation to tolerate great numbers of uninsured Americans might change. When this happens, the many years of effort will begin to be rewarded.

Although foundations might not have the power to change the larger forces that move America, the *Anthology* series shows that by targeting specific areas and making a commitment to them over many years, they can shape the direction of change once it begins happening. The challenge for the future is to develop a strategic vision where philanthropic resources can be brought to bear to increase Americans' access to health care at a time when market forces, rather than social values, predominate; when incentives to avoid serving chronically ill, isolated, and vulnerable people are inherent, and when an economic downturn threatens to increase the number of people without health insurance.

San Francisco Stephen L. Isaacs
Princeton, New Jersey James R. Knickman
August 2001 Editors

Notes

1. M. L. Berk and C. L. Schur, "A Review of the National Access-to-Care Surveys," *To Improve Health and Health Care 1997: The Robert Wood Johnson Foundation Anthology* (San Francisco: Jossey-Bass, 1997).

2. S. M. Allen and V. Mor, "Unmet Need in the Community: The Springfield Study," *To Improve Health and Health Care 1997: The Robert Wood Johnson Foundation Anthology* (San Francisco: Jossey-Bass, 1997).

3. J. R. Knickman, "Research as a Foundation Strategy," *To Improve Health and Health Care 2000: The Robert Wood Johnson Foundation Anthology* (San Francisco: Jossey-Bass, 1999).

4. Ibid.

5. S. L. Isaacs, L. G. Sandy, and S. A. Schroeder, "Improving the Health Care Workforce: Perspectives from Twenty-Four Years' Experience," *To Improve Health and Health Care 1997: The Robert Wood Johnson Foundation Anthology* (San Francisco: Jossey-Bass, 1997).

6. R. S. Frank, "The Health Policy Fellowships Program," *To Improve Health and Health Care: The Robert Wood Johnson Foundation Anthology, Volume V* (San Francisco: Jossey-Bass, 2002).

7. S. L. Isaacs, L. G. Sandy, and S. A. Schroeder, "Improving the Health Care Workforce: Perspectives from Twenty-Four Years' Experience," *To Improve Health and Health Care 1997: The Robert Wood Johnson Foundation Anthology* (San Francisco: Jossey-Bass, 1997).

8. L. G. Sandy and R. Reynolds, "Influencing Academic Health Centers: The Robert Wood Johnson Foundation Experience," *To Improve Health and Health Care 1998–1999: The Robert Wood Johnson Foundation Anthology* (San Francisco: Jossey-Bass, 1998).

9. T. Keenan, "Support of Nurse Practitioners and Physician Assistants," *To Improve Health and Health Care 1998–1999: The Robert Wood Johnson Foundation Anthology* (San Francisco: Jossey-Bass, 1998).

10. L. Bergeisen and J. C. Cantor, "The Minority Medical Education Program," *To Improve Health and Health Care 2000: The Robert Wood Johnson Foundation Anthology* (San Francisco: Jossey-Bass, 1999).

11. L. G. Sandy and R. Reynolds, "Influencing Academic Health Centers: The Robert Wood Johnson Foundation Experience," *To Improve Health and Health Care 1998–1999: The Robert Wood Johnson Foundation Anthology* (San Francisco: Jossey-Bass, 1998).

12. J. Firshein and L. G. Sandy, "The Changing Approach to Managed Care," *To Improve Health and Health Care 2001: The Robert Wood Johnson Foundation Anthology* (San Francisco: Jossey-Bass, 2001).

13. B. A. Stevens and L. D. Brown, "Expertise Meets Politics: Efforts to Work with States," *To Improve Health and Health Care 1997: The Robert Wood Johnson Foundation Anthology* (San Francisco: Jossey-Bass, 1997).

14. R. S. Frank, "The Health Policy Fellowships Program," *To Improve Health and Health Care: The Robert Wood Johnson Foundation Anthology, Volume V* (San Francisco: Jossey-Bass, 2002); and B. A. Stevens and L. D. Brown, "Expertise Meets Politics: Efforts to Work with States," *To Improve Health and Health Care 1997: The Robert Wood Johnson Foundation Anthology* (San Francisco: Jossey-Bass, 1997).

15. This phrase was used by Frank Karel, vice-president for communications of The Robert Wood Johnson Foundation, in "'Getting the Word Out': A Foundation Memoir and Personal Journey," *To Improve Health and Health Care 2001: The Robert Wood Johnson Foundation Anthology* (San Francisco: Jossey-Bass, 2001).

16. V. D. Weisfeld, "The Foundation's Radio and Television Grants, 1987–1997," *To Improve Health and Health Care 1998–1999: The Robert Wood Johnson Foundation Anthology* (San Francisco: Jossey-Bass, 1998).

17. M. S. Kaplan and M. A. Goldberg, "The Media and Change in Health Systems," *To Improve Health and Health Care 1997: The Robert Wood Johnson Foundation Anthology* (San Francisco: Jossey-Bass, 1997).

18. F. Karel, "'Getting the Word Out': A Foundation Memoir and Personal Journey," *To Improve Health and Health Care 2001: The Robert Wood Johnson Foundation Anthology* (San Francisco: Jossey-Bass, 2001).

19. D. Diehl, "The Emergency Medical Services Program," *To Improve Health and Health Care 2000: The Robert Wood Johnson Foundation Anthology* (San Francisco: Jossey-Bass, 1999).

20. S. Begley and R. P. Hearn, "Children's Health Initiatives," *To Improve Health and Health Care 2001: The Robert Wood Johnson Foundation Anthology* (San Francisco: Jossey-Bass, 2001).

21. M. Y. Holloway, "The Regionalized Perinatal Care Program," *To Improve Health and Health Care 2001: The Robert Wood Johnson Foundation Anthology* (San Francisco: Jossey-Bass, 2001).

22. J. Alper, "The Nurse Home Visitation Program," *To Improve Health and Health Care: The Robert Wood Johnson Foundation Anthology, Volume V* (San Francisco: Jossey-Bass, 2002).

23. P. Brodeur, "School-Based Health Clinics," *To Improve Health and Health Care 2000: The Robert Wood Johnson Foundation Anthology* (San Francisco: Jossey-Bass, 1999).

24. M. Y. Holloway, "Expanding Health Insurance for Children," *To Improve Health and Health Care 2000: The Robert Wood Johnson Foundation Anthology* (San Francisco: Jossey-Bass, 1999).

25. E. Bronner, "The Foundation and AIDS: Behind the Curve but Leading the Way," *To Improve Health and Health Care: The Robert Wood Johnson Foundation Anthology, Volume V* (San Francisco: Jossey-Bass, 2002).

26. C. Newbergh, "Tuberculosis: Old Disease, New Challenge," *To Improve Health and Health Care: The Robert Wood Johnson Foundation Anthology, Volume V* (San Francisco: Jossey-Bass, 2002).

27. D. J. Rog and M. Gutman, "The Homeless Families Program: A Summary of Key Findings," *To Improve Health and Health Care 1997: The Robert Wood Johnson Foundation Anthology* (San Francisco: Jossey-Bass, 1997).

28. I. M. Wielawski, "Reach Out: Physicians' Initiative to Expand Care to Underserved Americans," *To Improve Health and Health Care 1997: The Robert Wood Johnson Foundation Anthology* (San Francisco: Jossey-Bass, 1997).

29. S. Begley and R. P. Hearn, "Children's Health Initiatives," *To Improve Health and Health Care 2001: The Robert Wood Johnson Foundation Anthology* (San Francisco: Jossey-Bass, 2001).

⟞⟍⟍⟋⟍⟋⟍⟋⟍ Acknowledgments

The Robert Wood Johnson Foundation *Anthology* series is very much a team effort. We are fortunate to be working with such a talented group of people, most of whom have been together through all five volumes of the *Anthology*. We appreciate not only their high level of professionalism but also the degree of personal warmth that has made working together such a pleasure.

We would first like to acknowledge the singular contribution of Frank Karel. His vision helped launch the *Anthology* series, and he continues to offer his guidance, wisdom, insight, and good humor.

Since the first volume, each manuscript has been scrutinized by a panel of outside reviewers: William Morrill, Patricia Patrizi, and Jonathan Showstack. They make an invaluable contribution to every chapter and to the book as a whole.

The chapters are edited by C. P. Crow, an extraordinarily knowledgeable and gifted editor, and Molly McKaughan, who, as a writer and as co-director of the Foundation's grant-reporting unit, brings a unique perspective to the *Anthology*. Our thanks to both.

Within The Robert Wood Johnson Foundation, many people play an important role. We wish to thank Deborah Malloy for her tireless efforts in organizing materials—and people—at the Foundation; Sherry deMarchi for her willingness to be of assistance throughout the entire process; Linda Potts for her high level of professionalism in handling administrative matters; Paul Moran for stepping in so ably after Linda's retirement; Joseph Wechselberger, Carol Owle, and Carolyn Scholer for handling financial matters with such efficiency; Richard Toth and Julie Painter for assuring the accuracy of numbers pertaining to grant awards; Emily Snell for her research assistance; and Hinda Feige Greenberg for tracking down hard-to-find materials.

Many others have made a significant contribution. We would like to express our appreciation to Ty Baldwin, who enters editorial changes, and to Chris Chang, who is our fact checker. At Jossey-Bass, Andy Pasternack, the health series editor, and his colleagues Gigi Mark and Amy Scott handle production and distribution adroitly.

Various people reviewed the book, either in part or in whole. We thank Michael Beachler, Robert Campbell, Chris Conley, Ruby Hearn, Paul Jellinek, Nancy Kaufman, Terrance Keenan, Kate Kraft, Marion Ein Lewin, David Olds, Michael Rothman, Lewis Sandy, Steven Schroeder, Pauline Seitz, Warren Wood, and Judith Whang.

We would be remiss if we did not express our gratitude to each of the authors for the high quality of their work and for their patience in dealing with what must have seemed like endless queries from the editors.

At Health Policy Associates, we would like to thank Greta McKinney for handling the bookkeeping and financial reporting so efficiently and Elizabeth Dawson for shepherding the book through its final stages.

Finally, we owe a special debt to John Rodgers. John has excelled as a researcher, editor, and manager of the entire process from beginning to end. This will be John's last year as research and editorial associate for the *Anthology*; now he moves on to devote himself fully to health research. He has made an invaluable contribution, and he will be missed.

S.L.I.
J.R.K.

To Improve Health and Health Care

Volume V

Programs

CHAPTER ONE

~~~ The Nurse Home Visitation Program

Joseph Alper

Editors' Introduction

In this chapter, Joseph Alper, an award-winning journalist specializing in health care, examines nurse visitation programs. These programs arrange for nurses to pay regular visits to disadvantaged first-time mothers during and after their pregnancies to help them become better parents and to link them with social services and other support systems. They are the brainchild of David Olds, currently a professor of pediatrics, psychiatry, and preventive medicine at the University of Colorado Health Sciences Center.

Along with other foundations and the federal government, The Robert Wood Johnson Foundation funded a test of the idea in Elmira, New York, in 1978. When home visits by trained public health nurses appeared to improve the health of poor children and their mothers, the Foundation, among others, next funded a test in Memphis, Tennessee. Since then, Olds and others have demonstrated and tested variants of the concept at various locations around the country.

A number of lessons emerge from three decades of experience with nurse home visitation programs. First, evaluations of various approaches to home visits indicate that only the original model yielded unambiguously positive results. This raises an important issue: how close do replications of an innovative program have to be in order for researchers to consider the results the same as those of the original? A tension often arises between imposing a single model in diverse settings and letting individual communities bend a model to fit local circumstances. Nurse home visiting is one case where the model does not seem very bendable.

A second lesson is the importance of carefully testing a new service delivery idea before advocating its widespread adoption. Although the series of nurse home visitation experiments takes this idea to something of an extreme, a precise understanding of the strengths and limits of the approach would not have emerged without testing in a variety of circumstances. Moreover, the findings that did emerge influenced other Foundation-supported child development programs, such as the Infant Health and Development Program and the Urban Health Initiative, which were discussed by Sharon Begley and Ruby Hearn in last year's *Robert Wood Johnson Foundation Anthology.*

A third lesson is the value of foundations' sticking with an idea for a long time. The Robert Wood Johnson Foundation has nurtured the nurse home visitation program for almost three decades. The field has gained insights that would not have emerged with the three to five years of funding that normally characterizes grants from foundations.

I t was a rainy, cold October day in Oklahoma City as Margaret Black, a nurse in Oklahoma's Children First program, sat waiting in her car outside Yolanda Harris's home.[1] Yolanda, an 18-year-old high school senior, was running late for her appointment with Black, but the nurse was not surprised. "First, she's a teenager, and second, between school and being a mom, she's got a very full plate." Just then, a car pulled up to the worn-down house in one of Oklahoma City's poorer neighborhoods, and out bounded Yolanda carrying her school book bag over one shoulder and her nine-month-old son, Sierra, over the other. As she waved goodbye to the relative who had dropped her off, she said, "Sorry I'm late, but I had to talk to one of my teachers after school. Come on in."

It was time for Black's semi-monthly home visit with Harris, an obviously intelligent girl trying to cope with the demands of being both a first-time mother and a high-school student. Today's visit was supposed to focus on methods that parents can use to help their babies when they are crying inconsolably. Instead, Harris had other issues that needed immediate attention. "I have a new social worker and he's making me fill out more forms—again—before the day care center can get paid, and I'm afraid that I'm going to be dropped from the center," said Harris, who hopes to win a scholarship and attend college but is clearly upset by this new roadblock in her path. "And I also have to get my application form in so that I can take my ACTs."[2]

Black, who has been an inner-city public health nurse for two decades and has run into this situation before, calms the teenager and then asks her what she thinks she needs to do to resolve the situation. Harris finds a piece of paper and starts making a list. First, call the day care center and tell them that the paperwork is on its way. It will be the first time she's ever been late in filling out any forms for the day-care center, so it's unlikely that the center will drop her immediately. Second, get the ACT application in the mail by the deadline, which is the day after this particular visit. Third, find her copy of the forms she filled out previously and copy the information to the new forms. Fourth, do her homework. After making the list, Harris was in a brighter mood and was ready to talk to Black about her son and today's parenting lesson.

Though the discussion between the two women was interrupted frequently by the comings and goings of various people passing through the house, Harris was focused on the advice that Black was giving her. At the same time, she was keeping an eye on her very inquisitive son, who was intent on exploring everything in Black's bag. "Sierra, let me see that," she said as the boy picked up the weighing tray of Black's portable scale. With a big smile on his face, he handed it to her and then started to pull out the wooden alphabet blocks that Black brings with her as a diversion.

As the 90-minute visit came to a close, Black handed Harris some materials about nine-month-olds and commended her on how she handled both the current crisis and her son. Later, commenting to a visitor, the nurse said, "I'm proud of that girl. She has really benefited from this program, particularly in the way that she's learned how to solve problems on her own. She's become a strong parent, and she's doing a great job with her son under circumstances that would crush many new parents. And while nothing's certain in this world, I have a good feeling that she's going to make something of herself and that her son is going to do just fine."

⬩⟋⟍⟋⬩ Nurses Helping New Mothers Help Themselves . . . And Their Child

Yolanda Harris and her son are fortunate. "I don't know what I would have done without Mrs. Black's help, because I really didn't know how to be a mom, let alone how to be an adult," she said. "And I know that Sierra is getting a better start on life than I ever did."

That improved start is something that thousands of infants and toddlers nationwide have already received and tens of thousand more have an opportunity to get from their parents' involvement in programs that have grown out of a 20-year research and development project that has helped economically disadvantaged first-time mothers become better parents. By providing a better start to both parenthood and childhood, the Nurse Home Visitation Program[3] hopes to avoid some of the adverse consequences faced by many children born into less-than-optimal circumstances.

"Children of economically disadvantaged first-time mothers are more likely to be low-birth weight babies, more likely to be abused, more likely to live in a family where abuse occurs, more likely to get involved in juvenile crime, and are less likely to get the good parenting and developmental stimulation children need to live up to their fullest potential," said David Olds, who is currently a professor of pediatrics, psychiatry, and preventive medicine at the University of Colorado Health Sciences Center. He has been developing, testing, and refining the Nurse Home Visitation Program over the past two decades with continuing long-term support by The Robert Wood Johnson Foundation and grants from the U.S. Department of Justice, the U.S. Department of Health and Human Services, the National Institute of Mental Health, the Carnegie Corporation, the Commonwealth Fund, the David and Lucile Packard Foundation, the Ford Foundation, the William T. Grant Foundation, the Pew Charitable Trusts, and the Colorado Trust.

"By using trained nurses to provide a fairly intensive amount of training and instruction to mothers throughout pregnancy and during the first two years of a newborn's life, we hope to counteract many of these negatives and get mothers and their children pointed along a better path in life," Olds says.

The basic premises of Olds' work are that poor, first-time parents often lack the problem-solving and interpersonal skills that make for a good parent, and that an intensive program of regular visits, starting during pregnancy, by specially trained nurses can provide those skills. As a corollary, this approach can also give the mothers the intellectual resources to take charge of their own lives and better their circumstances, which in turn will also benefit their children.

"Most of the women who participate in this program are young, and don't have the financial resources or sense of direction to take good care of themselves or their babies," Olds said. "Therefore, our program places most of the emphasis on the mother—getting good prenatal care to start with, and then building on the idea that women will be better mothers and create a better environment for their child if they are armed with the skill and confidence that they can succeed, both as adults and as parents."

The purveyors of that skill and confidence are nurses, whom Olds considers to be the key to the program. "Not only do nurses receive extensive training in women's and children's health, but good nurses are also great at managing the kind of complex clinical situations that occur in at-risk families," he said.

There's another benefit to using nurses, too, according to Annette Jacobi, the director of Oklahoma's Children First program—the first statewide implementation of the Nurse Home Visitation Program. "We've found in Oklahoma that most women, and particularly poorer women, hold nurses in higher esteem than they do other professionals or paraprofessionals, and that works to the program's advantage, because it's so heavily grounded in teaching. That's not a knock on social workers or other professionals, but, rather, a credit to how mothers perceive the strengths of nurses. They are thought of as both caring and able to help pregnant mothers with their health concerns, and that's something that most women need as they learn to become parents."

The Nurse Home Visitation Program recruits public health nurses and provides them with extensive training in matters relating to maternal and infant development and teaching problem-solving skills to new mothers. The nurses are schooled on the program's home visitation protocols, which focus on five specific areas: personal health, environmental health, maternal role development, maternal life-course development, and family and friend support. The content of these protocols is organized to reflect the challenges which women are likely to confront at different stages of pregnancy and during the first two years of the child's life. The nurses are also trained in the various standard physical and emotional assessments, that they will use at each stage of the mother's and child's development over the two-plus years to spot any potential problems while they are still easily addressed.

During home visits, nurses carry out four major activities. First, they promote changes in behavior that will positively affect pregnancy, the health and development of the child, and maternal life course, or how the mother's life unfolds. Second, they help women build supportive relationships with family members and friends; such relationships help mothers feel that they are not alone in the world, but rather that they have a nurturing and caring support group that can help them through the inevitable times that try any parent. Third, they try to link family members with health and human services. Fourth, they perform a general health assessment of the child, which includes measuring the child's weight and height.

The nurses are trained to help with problems that come up, but to do so by guiding mothers to develop their own solutions. This helps prevent home visits from turning into gripe sessions, and keeps both nurse and parent from straying from the activities that need to occur. "There's always the opportunity to get too involved in the day-to-day problems families face, but the training stresses again and again the importance of coming back to the curriculum, to staying on-message," said Chris Russell, who is both a visiting nurse in the local Denver program and a trainer for the national Nurse Home Visitation Program office. "I think that's one of the keys to this program and one of the big differences from your more typical public health effort at home visiting."

—— A Program Built on Theory and Research

The Nurse Home Visitation Program began when David Olds was a graduate student in developmental psychology at Johns Hopkins University in Baltimore. "Inner-city Baltimore in the early 1970s was a rough place, and it was frustrating working with kids who had experienced so much trauma in their lives that what we were able to do for them was too little and too late," Olds said. "So when I got my Ph.D. I started thinking about how we could reach kids early and perhaps have a bigger positive influence on their lives. The conclusion I came to was that we needed to start with the mothers, to really focus on helping a mother be a better parent from the time her child was born."

Olds landed his first job as an assistant professor at the University of Rochester, and soon after arriving there he designed an experiment to test the hypothesis that working intensively with first-time mothers would benefit their children significantly. Olds set up the first test in Elmira, New York, a town of approximately 100,000 residents in a semi-rural Appalachian county. Funding for the ambitious project designed by an unknown assistant professor came from The Robert Wood Johnson Foundation. Program officers remember being impressed with both the scientific design of the experiment and the fact that the program had sound theoretical underpinnings.

The program Olds developed is grounded in theories of human ecology, self-efficacy, and human attachment. "Together, these theories suggest that behavior change is a function of a family's social context as well as an individual's beliefs, motivations, and emotion," Olds explained. "For example, human ecology theory emphasizes that a child's development is influenced by the type of care that the parents provide, and that, in turn, is influenced by characteristics of the family, its social networks, its neighborhood and community, and by the interrelations among them." As a result, the program trains nurses to enhance the material and social environment by involving other family members, including fathers, in the home visits and by linking families with needed health and human services.

Self-efficacy theory, on the other hand, provides a useful framework for understanding how women make decisions on their own, apart from their social support network, about their health-related behavior during pregnancy, the ways they care for their children, and how they approach their own personal development. According to Olds, self-efficacy theory implies that a woman's perceptions of her abilities can influence the choices that she will make and how much effort she will put into overcoming any obstacles she encounters.

Building on this idea, Olds designed the Nurse Home Visitation Program curriculum to help a woman understand what is known about the influence of particular behaviors on her health and on the health and development of her baby. In addition, the curriculum places a heavy emphasis on developing mothers' realistic goals and achievable objectives. The nurses help women recognize their successes in managing their lives and, through the acknowledgment of their small successes, help women develop the confidence that they can achieve their goals. Over the course of the program, such activities increase a woman's confidence in taking on ever larger challenges.

The third theoretical underpinning, which comes from the literature on attachment theory, stresses the importance of a child's biologically driven attachment to a few specific caregivers and the role of that attachment in developing a child's trust in the world and a capacity for empathy and responsiveness. The curriculum therefore emphasizes sensitive, responsive, and engaged parenting in the early years of a child's life. In addition, the nurses work hard to help mothers and other caregivers review their own childhoods and make decisions about how they wish to care for their children in light of how they were raised. The nurses also promote empathic, trusting relationships between the new mothers and other family members.

In April, 1978, armed with a curriculum designed around these basic tenets, Olds and his colleagues started training nurses and recruiting pregnant, first-time mothers-to-be in Elmira, New York. Over the next 30 months, their efforts resulted in 400 women being enrolled in the experiment; 62 percent of the women were unmarried, 48 percent were younger than 19 years of age, and 59 percent were poor. After stratifying the women by socioeconomic status, the researchers randomly assigned them to one of four groups. In the first group, 100 women received home visits from trained nurses during pregnancy. In the second group, 116 women received home visits during pregnancy and during the first two years of their children's lives.

There were two control groups. In the first control group, 90 women received no home visits from nurses and the children received sensory and developmental screening at ages one and two years. The second control group of 94 women also received no home visits but were given free transportation to regular prenatal and well-child visits, and their children, too, were screened at ages one and two.

Over the course of the experiment, nurses completed an average of nine visits during pregnancy and 26 visits in the two years after birth. Typically, nurses were scheduled to visit women once a week during the first month of enrollment, and then every other week until the baby was born. For women in the second group, weekly visits were scheduled for the next six weeks to help the mother and the newborn adjust, after which time visits occurred every other week until the baby was 21 months old. For the last three months, visits were monthly.

The results of this experiment were very promising, though only among low-income mothers. "For example, during pregnancy, nurse-visited women improved their diets and made a substantial cut in the amount they smoked," Olds said. "Their children were born with higher birth weights and the mothers made better use of local services and had a more extensive network of social support by the end of their pregnancy. We also saw an 80 percent drop in child abuse and neglect, which was a very nice surprise."

Follow-up studies found that subsequent pregnancies dropped 42 percent among women who had received the full course of nurse visits through the second year, while rates of high school completion and employment increased. "Evidently, the women were learning their lessons and taking steps to better their lives and the lives of their children," Olds said. One surprising finding was that middle-income women who had enrolled in the program showed very few benefits from the interventions in comparison to middle-income women in the control groups.

Fifteen years after the last woman graduated from the program, Olds and his colleagues from the University of Rochester, Cornell University, the University of Denver, and the University of Colorado revisited the children and found that the program had benefited these children in significant ways far beyond their toddler years. At the time of the assessment, the then-adolescent children had run away less than their peers who had been in the control groups, had fewer arrests, convictions, and parole violations, fewer sex partners, smoked fewer cigarettes per day, and drank alcohol less frequently. Their parents reported that the children had fewer behavioral problems related to the use of alcohol and drugs.[4]

"This is a remarkable finding," said Shay Bilchek, a former Justice Department official who oversaw youth violence prevention programs and who is now the executive director of the Child Welfare League of America in Washington, D.C. "It's one thing to see positive outcomes a year or two after an intervention, but to see these kinds of benefits 15 years later says to me that we as a nation should be putting the resources into making this program available to every low-income first-time mother in this country."

—— On to Memphis and Denver: Repeated Tests in Different Settings

Although the initial Elmira results were promising, Olds believed that his study, while well-designed, was limited by the population of women he had studied. "I firmly believed that we needed to replicate the Elmira work in a bigger, preferably urban area and in a different ethnic population," said Olds, who settled on Memphis and surrounding Shelby County as the next place to test the Nurse Home Visitation Program.

Besides using a different test population, the Memphis trial was designed to simulate what Olds considered to be a more "real-world situation." The study would rely on Memphis's system of public health nurses, who would receive training from Olds and his colleagues but would then administer the program with minimal input. An unexpected complication—a severe nursing shortage—led to high staff turnover, but this was the sort of problem that would affect the program if it ever expanded to a national scale.

The Memphis study began in June of 1990, and over the next 15 months 1,159 women who were less than 29 weeks into their pregnancy were recruited from the Regional Medical Center at Memphis. Enrollment was restricted to low-income mothers-to-be who met two of three criteria: they were unmarried, had not graduated from high school, or were unemployed. "We wanted to concentrate our resources on the highest-risk families," Olds explained. Once again, the women were stratified according to age, race, and income status, and were randomly assigned to a treatment or control group.[5]

Perhaps not surprisingly, given the less-controlled conditions, the results from the Memphis trial were not as overwhelmingly positive as they were in Elmira. On the plus side, women receiving home visits from nurses were healthier at the end of their pregnancies than those women in the control group, and children whose mothers received nurse visits suffered fewer injuries than did the children in the control group. Women receiving nurse visits also had fewer subsequent pregnancies, replicating the finding in Elmira.[6]

Unlike Elmira, the Memphis study did not find that the birth weight of newborns increased, and did not measurably reduce child abuse and neglect, probably because the rate of state-verified cases was too low—3 to 4 percent in the target population. Nor did it produce a significant drop in smoking, though this probably resulted from the fact that so few women in the Memphis trial smoked. In general, the improvements seen in the Memphis study were not as large as in the Elmira experiment. The most likely explanation for this is that the Memphis study did meet Olds' objective of representing a more real-life, less strictly controlled situation. "The fact that the Memphis study did replicate the meaningful reductions in childhood injuries that we saw in Elmira was very exciting, because it means we can allow some latitude in how the program is implemented and still expect positive results," Olds said.

This last point is particularly important. "What we've seen with many social programs aimed at improving parenting and child outcomes in at-risk populations, including some of the other home visitation programs, is that they work very well under hothouse conditions, where quality control is tight, where the developers are involved in every step of the implementation," said Ruby Takanishi, president of the Foundation for Child Development in New York City. "But when these programs enter the real world, we usually see that the outcomes are far less impressive. I think that's why the results from David Olds' work are so notable—there is enough quality control built into the program that it continues to generate positive outcomes in real world settings."

When reports on the Memphis study began appearing in the literature in the mid-1990s, they attracted the attention of many, including the Justice Department, who thought the results were strong enough to move the program out of the experimental stage. "We were quite impressed with the results on child abuse and maltreatment, because those are antecedents of adolescents getting involved in drugs and crime," Shay Bilchek said. "We secured funding under the auspices of Operation Weed and Seed and worked with David to set up six sites in high crime, inner-city settings, including Los Angeles, Oklahoma City, and Oakland, California."

At about the same time, Olds was setting up yet another trial, this time in Denver, where he had relocated to join the faculty at the University of Colorado School of Medicine. In 1993, the Colorado Trust had invited Olds to talk about the Nurse Home Visitation Program. Impressed with the plan, officials from the university recruited him to create the National Center for Children, Families and Communities, with the goal of disseminating this program to 100 communities.

But before embarking on a national dissemination effort, Olds wanted to run one more trial of the program, in Denver, both to refine the curriculum and training methods further and to test one important question—is it necessary to use nurses instead of trained paraprofessionals, which include certified nurses aides, community health care aides, physician assistants, and social workers? "Using nurses is expensive, and we wanted to address the criticism that we had heard that this program was too costly, that we could save money by using paraprofessionals without sacrificing efficacy," Olds said.

Preliminary results from the Denver randomized study, which ran from March of 1994 to June of 1999 and included 735 low-income first-time mothers, answered this criticism. Nurses were able to complete more visits than paraprofessionals, and the turnover among paraprofessionals was nearly twice that of nurses. In addition, paraprofessionals were less comfortable sticking to the defined home-visit guidelines and intervention strategies, a factor that would not bode well for obtaining the best outcomes.[7] Indeed, further analysis of the study data, which was presented in April 2001 at the Society for Research in Child Development meeting, has shown that nurse visits produced better outcomes than did paraprofessional visits.[8]

—⁓— Three Home Visiting Programs

There are, of course, other home visitation programs with similar aims—to improve the lives of children by giving them a better start on life. According to a 1999 report by the David and Lucile Packard Foundation on home visitation programs,[9] the number of young children served by such home programs more than doubled in the 1990s, from about 200,000 in 1993 to over 550,000 in 1999. "Much of this growth, we think, has resulted at least in part because of the well-documented findings of the Nurse Home Visitation Program research effort," said Deanna Gomby, deputy director of the David and Lucile

Packard Foundation's Children, Families, and Communities program and coauthor of the 1999 study.

Hawaii's Healthy Start Program

Hawaii's Healthy Start Program is the oldest continuing home visitation program. Started in 1975 as a single-site test on the island of Oahu, the program has now been adopted statewide with an annual budget of $6 million. It has also been modified and adopted by Healthy Families America, a home visitation program being disseminated by Prevent Child Abuse America, based in Chicago.

Healthy Start's goal is to identify vulnerable families before their day-to-day stresses, isolation, and poor parenting skills lead to abusive and neglectful behavior toward their children.[10] Trained paraprofessionals recruited from the community visit at-risk families for at least three years after the birth of their child. Visits are weekly at first and gradually decrease to quarterly as family functioning improves. Home visits focus on establishing trusting relationships with family members and then with imparting problem-solving skills. In addition, home visitors help families connect to various social services agencies when appropriate, and make sure that the children in the families receive appropriate medical care and nurturing parenting.

Evaluations of the first few Healthy Start projects were problematic. There were no control groups, for example. Nevertheless, abuse and neglect rates and stress levels among visited families were lower after the families participated in the program when compared to data from historical records. Even with these limited results, the Hawaii state legislature decided to expand the program statewide beginning in 1989.

With funding from The Robert Wood Johnson Foundation, the Annie E. Casey Foundation, the David and Lucile Packard Foundation, and the U.S. Department of Health and Human Services, the state conducted a more thorough, controlled evaluation of the program in 1994 and 1995. The evaluation found that the program was not implemented uniformly across the sites studied, retaining families in the program was difficult (attrition was as high as 50 percent after one year), and home visits rarely occurred as often as planned.

Although the effects of the program were modest after one year, at some sites the benefits increased in subsequent years. For example, mothers in the home visiting group were less likely to hold jobs at a one-year follow-up than were those in the control groups, but were more likely to be employed two years after completing the program. Overall, however, there were few differences between families who had received home visits and those in the control group who had not.

Healthy Families America

Before the results of the more thorough evaluation were in, Prevent Child Abuse America, with funding from the Ronald McDonald House Charities, decided to take Hawaii's Healthy Start Program and make it the basis of a nationwide effort to reduce child abuse in at-risk families. Thus in 1992 was born Healthy Families America, which is not so much a defined home visiting program as an initiative to help local communities create their own home visiting project based on some shared principles. "We're not a curriculum-based program," said Kathryn Harding, director of the National Center on Child Abuse Prevention Research, the research arm of Prevent Child Abuse America. "Instead, we help communities create their own programs based on 12 critical elements, such as the need for programs to start prenatally or when the child is first born and the need for services to be culturally relevant. In addition, our program stresses the importance of integrating the project with existing social support networks and social services organization in each community. We believe that the role of Healthy Families America is not to be an island but to enhance the existing service provider networks by adding a home visiting component."

While Olds stresses uniformity across program sites—staying faithful to the model—as a critical key to obtaining the best outcomes possible, Healthy Families America takes the opposite stance. "This is not a monolithic approach but, rather, a commitment to a set of principles," Harding said.

Because of that, evaluation of the program has been difficult. Harding's assessments have found that few of the programs actually follow the organization's guidelines or integrate themselves into the local public health systems in their communities. Despite this problem, some assessment has been possible. The program's effect on child abuse has been mixed. In some cases, the incidence of child abuse among mothers receiving home visits appeared lower than the rate for a comparable population, but other studies found no difference. More promising, however, is that participating families showed improvement in the quality of parent-child interactions and parental skills, and made more effective use of health care services.[11] "The nature of the Healthy Families America initiative has made it difficult to accurately assess the impact of the program, but I think the data we do have suggest that intensive home visiting does have a positive impact on families," Harding said.

The Parents as Teachers Program

Begun in Missouri in 1981, Parents as Teachers is a home visiting program whose goal is to have healthy, well-developed children who are ready for school. The program uses trained and certified parent educators—preferably educators, health care workers, and social workers—to make monthly visits, starting before, but no later than six months after, birth and continuing for the first three years of the child's life. The parent educators strive to increase parents' ability to nurture their children and prepare them for success in school. Group meetings supplement the home visits by allowing parents to share insights and build informal networks.

An assessment conducted by SRI International in Palo Alto, California, suggests that the Parents as Teachers program should be judged as popular but largely ineffective.[12] According to the study, parents did not show an increase in parenting knowledge or parenting attitudes despite these elements being the main focus of the program. There were, however, small but inconsistent advances in children's cognitive development; the children in the Parents as Teachers program may have enjoyed a little more than a month advantage over their peers who were not in the program. Children of Spanish-speaking Latina mothers, in particular, showed the most benefit from the program.

Since this evaluation was completed, the Parents as Teachers program has changed in several ways. The most significant change is the development of a new curriculum that reflects the latest research about how the brain develops during the first three years of life. The new curriculum, which will require more home visits by the certified parent educators, is based on neuroscience principles linked to infant and toddler development that have been translated into language that parents can understand and apply. It became the standard curriculum used by the Parents as Teachers program starting in 1999.

—— Limitations and Promise of Home Visitation

While it is hard to find fault with the good intentions that every home visitation program has at its core—to use home visitors to help improve the lives of at-risk children and their parents—it is equally difficult to deny the fact that the majority of these programs do not work as advertised. "Home visitation programs are really empty vessels into which you pour many, many different curricula and different philosophies of working with at-risk families," said the Packard Foundation's Gomby, who has spent a substantial amount of time over the past decade assessing these programs. "But aside from the work that David Olds has done, I think that most of these programs have neglected issues of implementation in real-world settings and of quality control in ensuring that the programs are actually carried out as designed. And that, I believe, is the biggest reason that we see the majority of these programs do so poorly when critically evaluated."

One problem, Gomby says, is that national program offices often put all of their resources into developing curricula and getting their programs adopted by various localities, and pay little attention to issues such as staff training and pay and how to retain families throughout the entire course of any given program. "Remember, these programs are trying to change people's lives with what amounts to at most 50 hours of contact spread out over a few years," Gomby said. "So when a significant number of the families don't even get that much attention, then perhaps it shouldn't be a surprise that the programs don't show much benefit."

In addition, assessments indicate that home visitation is not something that should be offered to all families, at least not with the goal of improving children's lives. "I think the data show that at best most of these programs are effective in helping only very narrow slices of the population, and, as such, we shouldn't be spending our limited resources trying to reach all women and all children who may be at risk," Gomby said.

That narrow slice, says Gomby, includes the most at-risk women and children: poor, single, and first-time mothers who often do not have access to the same social supports available to middle- and upper-income mothers. This is the very population that the Nurse Home Visitation Program serves and, in part, explains why it has been successful.

Gomby adds another reason. "The positive results that the Nurse Home Visitation Program generated show that when you work hard to maintain quality control, retain families in the program, and test various components of your program under rigorous conditions and then make changes when appropriate, you can have a measurable impact on the lives of children and their mothers," she concludes. "I think that it's also clear that we need to have realistic expectations about what these programs can accomplish. They are not a panacea, but they can make a difference when done right."

Olds wholeheartedly agrees with Gomby's remarks, "That's why we work so hard to make sure that the program is implemented correctly, that there's continual assessment and feedback to keep the local programs on track," he said. In fact, Olds and his colleagues have designed an internet-based information system to improve monitoring and provide more rapid feedback for local programs.

That is also why Olds has been reluctant to see the Nurse Home Visitation Program spread quickly. Four years ago, when the Oklahoma state legislature approached him about implementing the program statewide, he initially balked at the idea. But when it became clear that the state was going to proceed with or without his help, he reluctantly agreed to train the first group of nurses who would then act as trainers for the 240 nurses that Oklahoma planned to hire to blanket the state. Since then, he and his staff have kept close tabs on the program, providing regular feedback to help keep the effort on track and true to the curriculum.

What does Olds think of the program now? "Under the circumstances, they've done very well," he said. "Getting 240 nurses hired and trained and in place was an amazing feat, and I think the administrators' dedication to doing this right, to sticking to the curriculum, to maintaining quality control has been tremendous. I also think that the enormous amount of political support for the program and realistic expectations that people there have for the program have made it easier to do things correctly."

By the end of 2000, the 240 nurses in the Oklahoma program were seeing 7,000 clients, with hopes of adding a couple of thousand more women to the program. Annette Jacobi, the program director, believes that while it is still too early to tell if the program has had a positive impact on children, it is getting good results in terms of reducing smoking among pregnant women and problem pregnancies overall. "We also think we're seeing a drop in abuse and neglect among our clients, but we haven't had the positive effect we'd hoped for in terms of reducing subsequent pregnancies," she said. In addition, she said, the program has had a difficult time getting Native American women to participate.

Despite Oklahoma's success in getting its program up and running quickly, Olds would rather see states follow the 10-year adoption timetable set by Colorado. "I think that rapid dissemination should be, and will be, the exception rather than the rule, if for no other reason than most states won't have the resources to commit to ensure a high quality of implementation over a short time frame," Olds said.

One thing Colorado does share with Oklahoma is good political support for the program. But while that support came directly from the legislature in Oklahoma, it has been a grassroots effort—led by a group of lawyers—that is driving the process forward in Colorado. Jennifer Atler, a former corporate lawyer who gave up the boardroom to become director of the Denver-based nonprofit organization Invest in Kids, says her organization exists to spearhead the local adoption of what in Colorado is called the Nurse-Family Partnership program. "Believe it or not, a group of lawyers and other concerned citizens became aware of David's work and were so impressed that we formed Invest in Kids to build local support for this amazing program," Atler said.

Atler and her colleagues worked hard on two fronts: convincing the state's governor and legislature to commit funds from its share of the national tobacco settlement, and to generate local interest and support for the program. By all appearances, they were successful. Colorado made a commitment to increase funds for the program steadily through 2008 when the amount will reach $17 million—19 percent of the state's tobacco settlement funds in that year. The plan is to add between three and five new sites annually to the base of twelve sites that existed in 2000.

—— Lessons Learned

The problems facing poor first-time mothers, many of them single, at times seem so large as to be insurmountable, and it is alarming that so many programs designed to help these women and their children do not produce the intended results. Yet the trial in Elmira, and to a lesser degree the Memphis trial, found benefits for the mothers and children receiving nurse home visits. As Olds and his colleagues disseminate this program nationwide, with substantial funding from The Robert Wood Johnson Foundation, there are a number of important lessons to be learned from the successes and failures of home visitation programs.

QUALITY CONTROL IS ESSENTIAL FOR SUCCESS. Too many programs that work well in carefully controlled academic settings fail when transferred into the world at large, primarily because local implementations do not remain true to the original program design. One of the strengths of the Nurse Home Visitation Program has been the insistence of the program's developers that every community must follow the curriculum with only some room for adaptations that reflect local issues. Using a system of monitoring and regular feedback helps programs keep their nursing staff on target.

YOU GET WHAT YOU PAY FOR.   The most positive results from any home visitation program have come when nurses are the home visitors. Yes, nurses are the most expensive home visitor option, but the available data from a randomized, controlled trial indicate that mothers and children visited by nurses experience more positive gains than they do when the visitors are trained paraprofessionals.

CONTROLLED, RANDOMIZED TRIALS OF HOME VISITATION PROGRAMS MUST BE A CRITICAL COMPONENT OF ANY DEVELOPMENT WORK. Retrospective analyses of many home visitation programs have failed to show much, if any, positive effect on the lives of mothers and their children. According to the authors of these assessments, the lack of scientifically designed and implemented trials has hindered meaningful analysis.

POLITICAL SUPPORT IS CRUCIAL.   Home visitation is an intensive—and potentially intrusive—means of intervening in the lives of at-risk families, and as such it must have strong support in local communities. Building that support may take time and a substantial amount of effort, but it invariably eases the adoption of such programs. Good grass-roots political support also translates into realistic expectations for these programs.

Notes

1. "Yolanda Harris" is a pseudonym.
2. The ACT Assessment is a curriculum-based test for admission to college and university and an alternative to the SAT.
3. The Nurse Home Visitation Program is now called the Nurse–Family Partnership.
4. D. Olds, C. R. Henderson, Jr., R. Cole, J. Eckenrode, H. Kitzman, D. Luckey, L. Pettitt, K. Sidora, and J. Powers, "Long-term Effects of Nurse Home Visitation on Children's Criminal and Antisocial Behavior: 15 Year Follow-up

of a Randomized Controlled Trial," *Journal of the American Medical Association*, October 14, 1998, volume 280, number 14, pp. 1238–1244.

5. H. Kitzman, D. L. Olds, C. R. Henderson, C. Hanks, R. Cole, R. Tatelbaum, K. M. McConnochie, K. Sidora, D. W. Luckey, D. Shaver, K. Engelhardt, D. James, and K. Barnard, "Effect of Prenatal and Infancy Home Visitation by Nurses on Pregnancy Outcomes, Childhood Injuries and Repeated Childbearing," *Journal of the American Medical Association*, August 27, 1997, volume 278, number 8, pp. 644–652.

6. Ibid.

7. J. Korfmacher, R. O'Brien, S. Hiatt, and D. Olds, "Differences in Program Implementation Between Nurses and Paraprofessionals Providing Home Visits During Pregnancy and Infancy: A Randomized Trial," *American Journal of Public Health*, December 1999, volume 89, number 12, pp. 1847–1851.

8. D. Olds, R. O'Brien, D. Luckey, S. Hiatt, and C. Henderson, "Comparison of Pregnancy and Infancy Home Visitation by Nurses versus Paraprofessionals: A Randomized Controlled Trial," paper presented at the 2001 Biennial Meeting of the Society for Research in Child Development in Minneapolis, Minnesota, on April 19, 2001.

9. D. S. Gomby, P. L. Culross, and R. E. Behrman, "Home Visiting: Recent Program Evaluations—Analysis and Recommendations," *The Future of Children*, Spring/Summer 1999, volume 9, number 1, pp. 4–26.

10. J. D. Gray, C. A. Cutler, J. G. Dean and C. H. Kempe, "Prediction and Prevention of Child Abuse and Neglect," *Journal of Social Issues*, January 1979, volume 35, number 1, pp. 127–139.

11. D. A. Daro and K. A. Harding, "Healthy Families America: Using Research to Enhance Practice," *The Future of Children*, Spring/Summer 1999, volume 9, number 1, pp. 152–176.

12. M. M. Wagner and S. L. Clayton, "The Parents as Teachers Program: Results from Two Demonstrations," *The Future of Children*, Spring/Summer 1999, volume 9, number 1, pp. 91–115.

CHAPTER TWO

~~~ Tuberculosis: Old Disease, New Challenge

Carolyn Newbergh

Editors' Introduction

Tuberculosis remains the largest single infectious cause of death in the world. Each year, 8 million people worldwide contract the disease, and 2 million people die. Fully one-third of the world's population—most of them living in developing countries—are believed to be infected with the tuberculosis bacillus. Ten million Americans are thought to be infected, but only one in ten will ever become sick.[1]

While tuberculosis had been brought under control in the United States by the 1970s, it reappeared surprisingly in many areas of the country in the early 1990s. Concentrated largely among low-income populations, it coincided with the spread of AIDS. There was concern that it might reach epidemic proportions. The chronically underfunded public health systems in most cities had difficulty in mounting effective treatment and prevention efforts.

When a major health problem arises, there always is pressure for a large health care philanthropy like The Robert Wood Johnson Foundation to get involved in some way. Even modest Foundation support can increase awareness about a problem and signal the importance of the issue to those in the health field. Such was the case with the Foundation's involvement in trying to contain the spread of tuberculosis. Even though the Foundation tended in those years not to work on specific diseases, the special circumstances led the staff to develop a national program, Old Disease, New Challenge, and several single site initiatives.

The account of the Foundation's grantmaking in this area—by Carolyn Newbergh, a free-lance journalist specializing in health care issues—indicates that the results of the Foundation's efforts were mixed. Moreover, the spread of the disease was contained by other forces, and the feared epidemic never developed. Thus, it is difficult to make the case that the Foundation had a large impact. As one player involved in the initiatives reported, the Foundation dipped a "little toe" in the water. However, the Foundation learned some lessons from Old Disease, New Challenge about serving very difficult-to-reach populations such as migrant farmworkers, laborers crossing the United States-Mexican border, and poor people living in inner cities. The lessons might become even more relevant if the globalization of diseases leads to another resurgence of tuberculosis in this country.

—◦◦◦—

I t's hard to imagine that tuberculosis is the No. 1 infectious killer of all time. Today, when we live in fear of modern plagues like AIDS and Ebola, tuberculosis can seem a distant history lesson, a scourge of our grandparents' and great-grandparents' day but not ours. Yet the story of this disease is not done. With its remarkable ability to reappear when opportunity beckons, tuberculosis continues to challenge humanity, putting everyone who breathes air at risk.

Tuberculosis is truly an ancient sickness. Researchers have found signs of its origin in soil 15,000 years ago. Evidence of tuberculosis has been detected in the skeletal remains of Egyptian mummies from 4,400 years ago. The Greeks called this disease that slowly ate away at the lungs *phthisis*, for wasting away, because its pale sufferers progressively lost weight, appearing to wilt. Persistent low fevers and coughs that frequently brought up blood were other hallmarks of the disease, which mostly attacks the lungs. Over time, it became known as consumption and the white plague.

As Europeans started living in tighter groupings in cities, particularly during the Industrial Revolution, the disease became more menacing, rising to epidemic status. And it then became forever linked with the conditions of poverty that foster its spread—overcrowded housing, poor sanitation, and malnutrition. The white plague caused one-seventh of all Europeans' deaths in the nineteenth century.

For a time, the disease came to be regarded as an affliction of romantic geniuses, and it took many brilliant artists into its clutches—Chopin, Keats, Chekhov, Poe, Shelley, Charlotte and Emily Bronte.

Speculation abounded for years about what caused this sickness—was it the soil, bad air or climate, a tumor, heredity? Then, in 1882, a German country doctor, Robert Koch, identified the tuberculin bacillus, *Mycobacterium tuberculosis*, that causes the disease. This discovery led to the understanding that tuberculosis is contagious—caught through prolonged exposure to droplets in the air when someone with tuberculosis coughs, sneezes, laughs, or even talks—and set off intense scientific research to find a cure.

At the same time, a number of new treatment practices were being developed, with some success: collapsing a lung or a diseased cavity, removing ribs to deflate a lung, and cutting out damaged parts of a lung. By the twentieth century, many tuberculosis patients retreated to sanatoria in Europe and the United States, where they were quarantined for up to two years. The "cure" consisted of fresh, often cold, air, healthy food, and rest. Sanatoria slowed the spread of tuberculosis mostly by keeping contagious people away from the healthy. Although many patients recovered, it's not clear whether sanatoria improved long-term patient survival.

Major medical breakthroughs beginning in the 1940s heralded a new era. One drug after the next was discovered that could destroy the bacteria. Now people were truly restored to health, no longer having to give up jobs and family lives to reside at the sanatoria.

Effective drug treatment meant that tuberculosis's days as a virtual death sentence were over. In 1907, tuberculosis was the country's reigning killer disease, taking 156,000 lives, but 40 years later this scourge ranked seventh, with a death toll of 60,000. More remarkable progress would come: From 1953 to 1984, the number of active tuberculosis cases declined 5 to 6 percent a year, down from 84,304 to 22,201—a 74 percent drop.[2]

As people became confident that tuberculosis was being eradicated, fear of catching it faded away. With the threat seemingly over, efforts to stay on top of the disease ended. Government funding for programs that monitor, control, and treat tuberculosis were reduced to nothing in 1972. In its place, states received block grant money to use as they chose. Treatment shifted from hospitals, which no longer maintained isolation rooms to control contagion, to outpatient clinics. And by 1989 the U.S. Department of Health and Human Services' Advisory Council for the Elimination of Tuberculosis optimistically called for tuberculosis to be eliminated in the United States—less than one case per 1 million people—by the year 2010.[3]

But the optimism proved to be ill-founded, and tuberculosis staged an awful comeback. It began showing up in increasing numbers of people in the late 1980s and early 1990s—and this time in a more virulent form. From 1985 to 1992, the trend was unmistakable: the annual number of cases grew from 22,201 to 26,673—a 20 percent climb.[4] Tuberculosis was no longer receding into the past or solely the problem of developing countries with poor infection control. In New York, cases skyrocketed, and outbreaks in prisons and hospitals evoked age-old fears.

The biggest trigger for this tuberculosis resurgence was the human immune deficiency virus that causes AIDS. Ordinarily, about 90 percent of people who are infected with tuberculosis will show no signs, and the disease will be latent and noncontagious in them for the rest of their lives. But 10 percent of those who are infected will become ill with an active form of the disease, half of them within a year and the others usually when they are older and their immune system is weaker. With HIV, the immune system is so compromised that tuberculosis infection proceeds to active disease quickly, often within two months. And, in another deadly twist, tuberculosis speeds up HIV's disease progression, leading to death more rapidly. In fact, it is the foremost cause of death for people with HIV.[5]

This new epidemic had another ominous characteristic—drug resistance. Ordinarily, tuberculosis patients were treated for six to twelve months with four medications, because resistance to one drug wasn't uncommon. But now patients were showing up with bacteria that didn't respond to two or more of the most effective, least costly drugs that also cause the fewest side effects—usually to isoniazid and rifampin, the workhorses of the tuberculosis medicine cabinet.

This necessitated treatment with second-line drugs, which would take two years or longer, cost more, create other health problems, and might not cure the patient. Caring for someone with multiple-drug resistant tuberculosis can be 100 times as costly as for someone with a regular strain of the disease, reaching $250,000 for the medications and likely hospitalization; treatment for regular tuberculosis ranges from several hundred to a few thousand dollars.

And someone with tuberculosis of the multiple-drug resistant sort could spread this lethal form of the disease to others.

Ironically, the resistance develops from the nature of tuberculosis treatment. Patients with regular tuberculosis must swallow from four to 12 pills a day—a task people might give up on once they started feeling better in a few weeks. That's what was happening. But failing to complete the medication can lead to a relapse and, even worse, can allow the tuberculosis bacteria to mutate into a form that no longer responds to the medications that are taken.

The disease was preying mostly on poor and vulnerable people living at society's fringes—the homeless, people living with AIDS, migrant workers, alcohol and drug abusers, the incarcerated, and immigrants—people who are more likely to stop taking the pills prematurely. These individuals tended to be unattached to any medical system and lacked the social support to help them stick to a long course of therapy.

This combination of factors was not just a peril in the United States. Worldwide, the same trends were unfolding and in much greater numbers in developing areas such as sub-Saharan Africa and Asia, which lacked adequate health care systems, and in the jails of Russia, where the health infrastructure was in tatters. A 1991 article in the British medical journal *The Lancet* alerted readers that the intertwining of AIDS and tuberculosis amounted to one of the greatest public health disasters since the bubonic plague.[6] And in 1993 the World Health Organization declared tuberculosis a world health emergency.

As this wave of fear swelled, The Robert Wood Johnson Foundation decided to address the tuberculosis crisis. The Foundation, which at the time didn't direct grant money to specific diseases, made an exception for tuberculosis because of the threat that multiple-drug resistance posed. In 1993, the Foundation funded a three-year $6.65 million program called Old Disease, New Challenge: Tuberculosis in the 1990s designed to test innovative models for reducing barriers to health care among the people most at risk for tuberculosis. "This was a little toe in the water, to see what worked," said Nancy Kaufman, a vice-president of The Robert Wood Johnson Foundation. "This was a time when a crisis was looming, and it was important to be concerned. It was an opportunity to elevate, which we do with our name and money, the seriousness of this issue, and to be a stimulus."

Five demonstration projects around the country were chosen. The sites were Atlanta, Baltimore, New York City, North Florida, and San Diego.

The projects—directed toward the hard-to-reach, the disaffected urban poor, migrant workers, and people who cross the border with Mexico—were to incorporate collaborations among local government, medical schools and hospitals, and community-based organizations. They would screen for latent and active disease. Most would use directly observed therapy, a method of insuring that patients complete their medications by having someone observe them swallow their pills each day. This approach was just beginning to gain acceptance at the time, and today is standard practice. The use of culturally sensitive outreach workers would be crucial to the success of the program. The funding also included smaller grants for related tuberculosis projects such as forecasting how the epidemic was likely to progress and examining the ethical issues that tuberculosis raised.

In an unusual approach, anthropologists were hired to do a "qualitative evaluation." They were to "live" with the projects in the field and, by using extensive participant observation and interviews, get a close-up view of the workings of each project. They were to feed insights back to the project so changes could be made. As it turned out, their reports gave textured accounts of the various players and how they carried out their goals.

~~~ The New York City Project

To hear Danita Evans tell it, Bellevue Hospital's fight against tuberculosis was filled with glory days. A number of social service agencies that serve the poor would skin-test their clients for tuberculosis, and Evans and several other community liaison workers would whisk those who came up positive to Bellevue by subway or taxi. There she slashed through the red tape that ordinarily overwhelms the dispossessed people who were at the heart of the tuberculosis epidemic in the 1990s.

Patients no longer had to slog through the registration and appointment processes, which in the past had sometimes meant waiting a month to see a doctor. Evans got them a clinic card, a doctor's appointment, and the services they needed—all in one day. She shepherded them through getting an X-ray, a blood test, a sputum smear, and a doctor's evaluation. If left alone, she feared, these alienated, out-of-their-element patients, many of them substance abusers, homeless, mentally ill, or living with HIV, would find the hospital system too daunting and leave.

Evans worked with a passion stoked by the grim reality that New York City was the epicenter for this comeback epidemic in the United States, and that these people at society's margins were its favored prey. "It was like a rush for me," she says. "I'd get in the taxi, have three patients in back with me, many who hadn't been in one for a long time. It was exciting because I'd get the patients to Bellevue quickly. And I found that once I got hold of patients, they were mine. They'd come back for treatment."

Community liaison workers like Evans were at the heart of The Robert Wood Johnson Foundation project at Bellevue Hospital. The Shared Responsibility Program for Tuberculosis Casefinding and Treatment was conceived to try a new approach to getting the disaffected poor people most in danger of catching tuberculosis to trust an institution they had stayed away from in droves.

Bellevue, the oldest existing public hospital in the country, has a mission to serve the poor, and started the nation's first tuberculosis clinic

in a public hospital 100 years ago. By the 1990s, this 1,242-bed academic facility, affiliated with New York University, was thought of as too
big, imposing, and unreceptive to the very people who most needed it.
Many people couldn't cope with navigating this rambling building with
rules and regulations that seemed designed to keep them out.

At this time, active tuberculosis cases had climbed from the city's
all-time-low of 1,307 in 1978 to 3,811 in 1992—a case rate that translates to 50.4 per 100,000 people. One-quarter of them had the drug-
resistant forms of the disease. City residents were alarmed and
frightened as they learned of tuberculosis outbreaks in group-living
settings like prisons and hospitals and among health care workers. "In
places like Harlem, the case rate was 250 per 100,000 population,
which was incredibly high," said Neil Schluger, a co-principal investigator for the project who headed Bellevue's Chest Service.

With its long commitment to caring for tuberculosis patients,
Bellevue was again a major player. In 1992, the hospital carried the
largest active tuberculosis caseload in the state, with 511 newly diagnosed patients. Moreover, many of the patients didn't respond to more
than one of the most effective drugs, and the hospital had the highest
caseload of patients with both HIV and tuberculosis in the country.

To address the public health crisis and attract hard-to-reach
patients, Bellevue proposed a collaboration with five well-established
community-based organizations on the Lower East Side: the Lower
East Side Services Center, the Educational Alliance, the BRC Human
Services Corporation, Housing Works, and the Community Health
Project. These agencies met many of the needs of the people at risk,
and could connect them to Bellevue's tuberculosis program. Their
wide range of services included sheltering the homeless, providing
food, and treating substance abusers and people with HIV/AIDS.

"Our clients are a population that's well advertised but not well
served," said Ronald Williams, a program director at BRC, which provides residential and outpatient treatment for clients with substance
abuse problems, many of them homeless and mentally ill, and referrals to other services. "People at Bellevue had automatic attitudes
about our clients, because they could tell they were using. Our clients
didn't fit the nice-client mode and got pushed away. But when Danita
Evans walked the same patient through, he became a real person,
someone they'd actually look at and deal with."

The idea was that the community-based organizations would give
skin tests and questionnaires assessing tuberculosis risk to all of their

clients; those with positive tests or suspicious symptoms such as a persistent cough would go to Bellevue for chest X-rays, further testing, and evaluations. Those with active disease would be put on directly observed therapy, the supervised taking of pills. Preventive medication would be given to some with latent disease, but it would not be observed. The community liaison workers would be the bridge between Bellevue and the organizations, making sure that patients got appointments and kept them, were fully assessed, and then followed through with their treatment if one was given.

For the most part, this project clicked.

The project was led by hospital administrators who believed in it and took pains to bring it to life. Instead of telling the service agencies how the project would work, the hospital administrators invited them to help design the program. David Cohen, then Bellevue's medical director, provided strong leadership.

"We tried as much as we could to have these community-based organizations be equal to us in their input into the program," Schluger said. "We felt we had a lot to learn from them. These clients have all kinds of medical and social needs, and they're all equally important. You can't do much about one if there's a problem with the other."

The agencies let Bellevue know that many patients would feel insecure in a large institution that was new to them and, if faced with too many roadblocks on the way to the chest clinic, would simply give up. The project set out to remove barriers for these clients. The project's manager, Naomi Wolinsky, bent many hospital rules to blaze a new and truly easy way for these tuberculosis patients to get served expeditiously. She arranged for two chest clinic appointments to be set aside each day for the project's patients, insuring that they would almost always be seen.

Because of Wolinsky's efforts, the community liaison workers were able to get patients a chest clinic card quickly and escort them through the security guards and registration offices that would have discouraged them in the past. The workers were with the clients every step of the way, even giving them lunch and showing them where the restrooms were. They also provided tuberculosis education to the agencies and trained them to administer the purified protein derivative, or PPD, skin tests.

Those who were treated for tuberculosis were given an incentive to keep returning for the long course of directly observed therapy. After completing the first month, they would get 10 subway tokens each week that they kept their appointments.

The hospital allowed each agency to define how its relationship would work. In some cases, Bellevue gave funding directly to an agency. The agency's own staff member would function as the liaison worker, administering skin tests and escorting clients through the Bellevue maze. This occurred, for example, at the Educational Alliance, an agency with services for children, people with AIDS, substance abusers, and elderly people.

"You don't know how great it felt to do tuberculosis right," said Peter Cordero, the Educational Alliance's tuberculosis/AIDS coordinator who was also its community liaison worker. "If a patient was positive, we would take him to Bellevue for an X-ray and run interference for him. People feel very uncomfortable going to that place the first time." The Educational Alliance also provided tuberculosis education and screening to other local community organizations, particularly those serving Southeast Asian immigrants.

This project got some noteworthy results. Altogether, 3,828 people were evaluated, and 20 cases of active disease were found—representing a high tuberculosis rate of 522 cases per 100,000 population. Eight patients were diagnosed in each of the first two years of 1994 and 1995, four in 1996, and none in 1997, reflecting the nationwide decline in the epidemic.

Thirty-three percent of those who returned to have their skin tests read were found to be latently infected—1,163 people. From this group, 466 were further evaluated at Bellevue, and 55 were put on preventive therapy of isoniazid for six months; just 20 people completed it. Doctors viewed most of the clients as bad candidates for preventive medication because homeless people and drug addicts were unlikely to take pills for so long without directly observed therapy, which was not available to patients without active tuberculosis.

Schluger concluded that large-scale screening was worthwhile for finding active disease in a high-risk group such as this one and that treating those with tuberculosis through directly observed therapy had proven to be cost effective. At the same time, he determined that screening for latent tuberculosis as a way to prevent future cases doesn't make sense without treatment that includes directly observed therapy to insure that the drugs are taken to completion.[7] "We found that if all you were going to do is find latent tuberculosis without treating it, you have to think long and hard about whether this is how you should spend your dollars for tuberculosis control," Schluger said in an interview. "Are you doing everything else well before you focus on the latent cases?"

Nearly everyone involved applauded this project for creating a model that linked a big-city academic hospital with community organizations serving very difficult-to-reach populations and affording access to people with tuberculosis who might have gone untreated otherwise. In 1995, the project earned an honorable mention from the U.S. Department of Health and Human Services' Models That Work competition.

"It was an eye-opening experience," said William Rom, the Chest Service's current chief. "They got to street-level people we didn't know then. We got referrals and saw patients we wouldn't have seen otherwise."

The grant had some important side benefits as well: clients often complained of other health problems while at Bellevue and received treatment. Bellevue set up primary care clinics at some of the community organizations—such as pediatric and adult primary care clinics at the Educational Alliance. This was a plus both to the agency and to the hospital, which was looking to expand its revenue sources.

When Shared Responsibility drew to a close in 1997, the community-based organizations pushed for the services to continue, and administrators tried hard to find replacement funding. The New York City Department of Health agreed to fund two community liaison workers, including Evans, primarily to help more stable low-income people with latent infection get through directly observed preventive therapy, and to provide tuberculosis education.

But the scope of the liaison workers' job is much narrower today, and the chest clinic no longer reserves time slots for the agencies' clients. The community-based organizations lament that their agencies don't have a dedicated liaison like Evans and that they can no longer sail smoothly through Bellevue. In fact, few of them go there anymore. Most tuberculosis testing and treatment take place now through the Health Department anyway, but not that many clients go for the screening.

The Educational Alliance's Peter Cordero sometimes sends clients to Bellevue for skin testing, but he and Williams say the hospital is again regarded as an impenetrable institution. The registration process has been streamlined some for all patients, but not nearly enough for their clients. "I'm sorry to say it, but Bellevue has reverted to its byzantine method for dealing with patients," the BRC's Ronald Williams said.

Nevertheless, Bellevue soldiers on. Rany Condos, the Chest Service co-director and an assistant professor, says the hospital learned better how to meet the needs of the underserved. And even if it isn't tending to many of the agencies' clients, the Chest Clinic continues to offer directly observed therapy to active tuberculosis patients, directly observed preventive therapy for those with latent infections, and to provide isolation beds for those who are hospitalized.

And the community-based organizations say the program has had one important legacy: heightened tuberculosis awareness. "The first questions nurses here at BRC used to ask were whether you were in detox before and what drugs you use," Williams said. "Now they ask what drugs do you use and have you been tuberculosis tested. "

⁓ The San Diego–Tijuana Project

Pedro Perez sits in a modest Tijuana medical clinic, his navy sweats hanging loosely, his eyes cast downward as he speaks softly. It was 25 years ago, in 1975, that he first learned he had tuberculosis. He was driving a cab in Tijuana then, and he coughed a lot.

"I took the pills for a while until I stopped," Perez, 51 now, says somberly. He was feeling better and, he adds sheepishly, he really wanted a drink. Told that liquor and the tuberculosis medicines could be toxic to the liver, he chose alcohol.

When the cough flared up again, he returned for medical care. He was to repeat this starting and stopping routine five times, seeking treatment in Tijuana and just over the border in San Diego County, where he visited relatives from time to time. With all this interrupted treatment, the tuberculosis bacteria altered, and by his sixth attempt it no longer responded to the seven most effective medicines. And no other drugs were available in Mexico to cure his disease.

Perez was filled with despair—he coughed up blood, had feverish night sweats, was depressed, and feared for the health of the nine people living in his family home. Then he got a break. In 1994, his Tijuana clinic was able to obtain the pricey medications he needed through its new partnership with San Diego County as a demonstration site under the Old Disease, New Challenge program. Equally important, he received the kind of special treatment and support he desperately needed to see the treatment through. In the past, Perez had either been sent home with enough medicine for a month or with a prescription he sometimes couldn't fill.

Now a nurse watched to be sure he swallowed the pills each day, either at his home or at the clinic, and gave him a supply for the weekend. He was closely monitored and tested regularly. When at first he didn't improve, part of a diseased lung was removed and the drug treatment was resumed for 18 months. Family members received medicine to keep from becoming sick, too. This time, Perez said, he took his tuberculosis seriously and was cured.

"It if wasn't for this program and the effort put in, I know he wouldn't be here," his wife, Marcela Rodriguez says. "He was given so much attention from people here. We wished others could have a program that focuses on an individual's well being like this."

Perez's personal journey is a chilling introduction to the real people behind the global tuberculosis epidemic. The incidence of the disease and its drug-resistant form are highest in developing countries such as Mexico, where there is little or no directly observed therapy to help with adherence, and there are none of the drugs patients need when the most common ones no longer work.

For San Diego County, the world tuberculosis crisis was very close to home—virtually spilling over the backyard fence. In 1992, San Diego County's new tuberculosis case rate spiked up 75 percent, even higher than California's own alarming 45 percent rise. About 44 percent of the patients were Latino, two-thirds of them from Mexico.[8] Baja California, where Tijuana is located, had the highest active tuberculosis rate of the six Mexican border states. The county was finding—and still does find—that 20 percent of its tuberculosis patients were resistant to first-line medications. Drug resistance was even higher in Tijuana, at 30 percent, according to a 1994 study.[9]

"The need to do something was so obvious, because people cross this border more than 65 million times every year," said Alberto Colorado, who today is the county's binational coordinator. "There is constant movement and constant risk of exposure. These are people who take care of our children, our yards, serve food at McDonald's, work in the malls, movies, the racetrack, run the buses, visit family. For public health reasons, we need to understand that there are now more international interactions among people."

With a sense of urgency, San Diego County designed a program called A Model for Cooperation: U.S.–Mexico Tuberculosis Control.

It would become the Foundation's first binational program, and the most problem-riddled of the Old Disease, New Challenge grants.

Ambitious goals were set: to cure patients with regular and multiple-drug resistant tuberculosis and lower the number of new infections; to ensure that patients continued to receive medications when they crossed the border; and to educate people living in this high-risk area and their medical personnel about tuberculosis. The key to achieving the objectives would be beefing up the Tijuana clinic and developing a model for directly observed therapy there.

"The challenge in Mexico, the U.S., really everywhere in the world is not so much the diagnosis and getting medication," said Kathleen Moser, county tuberculosis control chief and the grant's principal investigator. "It's once a person is diagnosed and on medication, insuring that they take the medication the right way every day for six to nine to 12 months or more. The missing piece at that time in Tijuana was completion of therapy, and that's the ballgame."

The county subcontracted for services with two health clinics frequented by people who live and work in the border region: the San Ysidro Health Center, just two miles over the border into the United States, and the Centro de Salud Urbano, the downtown Tijuana public health clinic where Perez was treated.

A more modest binational collaboration between the San Ysidro clinic and the Centro de Salud Urbano had been running since 1984. Led by Benjamin Sanchez, a physician who would later become part of the new project's team, it was funded by the federal government. Under the new program, the United States government would continue to fund medicines and testing of sputum cultures, and The Robert Wood Johnson Foundation would cover the outreach with directly observed therapy to all patients and the very expensive medications for patients with multiple-drug resistant tuberculosis.

The two clinics would conduct tuberculosis screening, diagnosis, treatment, and directly observed therapy for patients with active disease and latent infection. They would also call ahead when they knew a patient was crossing the border to help insure the continuation of treatment.

The San Ysidro–Tijuana partnership had a number of pluses. It treated 170 patients, with about 75 percent completing treatment— an improvement over Tijuana's track record, which was estimated at 50 percent. The program put 20 of the patients with multiple-drug resistant tuberculosis in Tijuana on medications. Half of them completed the long regimen, which can take more than two years.

The project also allowed experimentation with approaches to stanching this disease that hadn't been seen before in Tijuana. Each day, two nurses and a social worker drove all over the city to visit patients, watch them take their pills, and monitor their progress. Additionally, they drove to people's homes to inform them they had active tuberculosis and searched for patients' close friends, co-workers, and other regular contacts so they could skin test them. (As it turned out, this was an arduous, time-absorbing process, and the project staff concluded that the model of delivering directly observed therapy was too inefficient and expensive.) Another benefit was the training of Tijuana and San Ysidro clinic personnel in the latest standards for tuberculosis screening, treatment, and infection control—an educational opportunity staff members say continues to pay dividends. The Tijuana clinic was also given sorely needed diagnostic equipment—an X-ray machine, a film-processing unit, and a small, separately ventilated sputum induction booth where patients who had difficulty producing enough sputum for a sample could cough without spreading bacteria to others nearby. And an informal referral system developed in which project staff members would at times call ahead to one another when a patient was relocating across the border and needed follow-up attention.

The project also ran into problems that severely limited its impact. Today, a sadness lingers as participants tell of the misunderstandings and the bitterness that overtook them. They attribute the discord largely to the difficulties inherent in bringing two countries of differing resources and cultures together.

Leadership was a major shortcoming. The grant burned through two overall project managers, both based at San Ysidro, who were viewed as out of their depth. The first manager was slow to iron out basic yet complex startup issues—how to pay workers in Tijuana and buy and transport equipment, two cars, medical specimens, and medication over the border. And both managers never addressed a crucial issue—that many of the San Ysidro staff members were uncomfortable providing tuberculosis services because they feared for their own health and legal risk to the clinic if other patients caught the disease. As a result, commitment to the project was never solid. And the second project manager created serious personnel problems at the clinic that led to tension, bad morale, and disrupted service before he finally left.

Financial disagreements also plagued the project. Both clinics involved in early project planning had contracts with the county that spelled out that they would be paid for delivering certain services. As it turned out, both clinics believed they should have gotten grant money to use as they saw fit, and ill will resulted as they waited instead to be given money to cover specific expenses and were told what to do. The Tijuana staff viewed this as a rich country dictating the rules to a poor one, leaving it no better off in the end.

"The feeling at the Tijuana clinic was 'Where is the money,'" said Benjamin Sanchez, the project's coordinator. "And they had a different idea of how the money should be spent. They even stopped collaborating with us at the end because of this. They said that they weren't getting the money so they wouldn't do anything." Anger and resentment worsened when the peso was devalued and project nurses working at the Tijuana clinic, who were paid in American dollars, earned seven times as much as the clinic's own nurses. "To this day, they say it undermined the whole tuberculosis control effort in Baja California, which is hard for me to understand," said Kathleen Moser, the project's principal investigator.

Most serious of all, though, San Ysidro's understanding of its mission was at odds with San Diego County's. At monthly case conferences, the county learned that San Ysidro was taking some tuberculosis patients recommended for directly observed therapy by their doctors or the county health department off of it. The project covered this cost, and it's not clear why the clinic dropped these patients. It was speculated that the clinic wished to use its outreach worker differently. San Ysidro was also responsible for caring for close associates or contacts of its tuberculosis patients regardless of whether they had health insurance. However, San Ysidro referred uninsured contacts to the county's tuberculosis clinic, 15 miles north, increasing the chances that they might stop treatment. As a result of these disputes, the county relieved San Ysidro of its duties two years into the three-year grant, and took over caring for the patients at its own tuberculosis clinic and at another county clinic closer to the border.

Moser and other county officials don't deny that the breakdowns and turbulence stunted the project's effectiveness. But they say the conflicts and problems in getting started stemmed from the complexity of creating a binational program and the need to stay sensitive to cultural subtleties and differences. This project, they said, really needed far more time to find its way. In fact, having learned that sending outreach workers to patients' homes wasn't practical, the county asked the Foundation to extend the grant an extra year and use unexpended money to change the directly observed therapy model in Tijuana to one that was delivered by *promotoras,* health promoters from within the local community.

This request led to the bitterest chapter of this grant's story. "We felt our program was just beginning, and we were just starting to understand how the binational model could work better," Moser said. "It is so difficult to get something going involving international relations. Three years was way too short to start up something new and difficult like this." The Foundation said no to the extension requested. The project hadn't performed well, and it was time to cut the losses, said Marilyn Aguirre-Molina, the Foundation's program officer for the project at the time. "We had a lot of meetings on this program," Aguirre-Molina said. "It was not a decision made easily or routinely. But there was nothing there to build on. It would have been an extension to start almost from scratch."

Since the project ended, in 1996, the San Diego County tuberculosis rate has declined, as it has elsewhere in the nation. Drug-resistant tuberculosis continues at 20 percent of cases because of the influx of people from Mexico and Southeast Asia. In 1998 the World Health Organization counted Mexico among the 16 "trouble spot" countries that accounted for more than half of the people worldwide with the disease.

Despite the internal tribulations, the binational program did have some lasting benefits. The X-ray machine continues to be used in Tijuana, and expertise in tuberculosis control and management improved among health care providers. More important, relationships—and some trust—did develop among public health officials in the county and in Tijuana. Today, regular meetings on regional approaches to tuberculosis are held, and annual binational conferences that were started under the grant continue, attended by hundreds of officials from both countries.

As a result of the project, the state of California broadened the informal referral system by funding the Cure TB program out of San Diego County's binational tuberculosis coordinator's office. With an 800 number, Cure TB gives to health officials treatment information concerning about 100 active tuberculosis patients each year who move between the United States and Mexico. The project also inspired a Texas initiative called Ten Against TB, in which the 10 states of the

United States and Mexico that share the border work together on tuberculosis control.

Meanwhile, when the project ended, the Centro de Salud Urbano in Tijuana was left with lesser diagnostic and treatment options. "We miss those benefits for our patients," said Concepcion Corona, the beleaguered chest clinic director there. "We got used to having resources, and suddenly they were cut off and we were left alone."

The Tijuana clinic has an active caseload of 125 tuberculosis patients, which is still high, and a disturbing 10 percent of them are children. The clinic does no drug-susceptibility tests to determine whether a patient doesn't respond to certain drugs—a dangerous omission that certainly leads many patients to be treated with the wrong drugs and allows them to spread the disease. With no real directly observed therapy occurring, patients come to the clinic once a week for their pill supplies.

At this clinic where Pedro Perez was finally cured of tuberculosis, there is little hope for patients like him whose disease can't be cured with drugs obtainable there. Corona is sure that he would have more multiple-drug resistant tuberculosis patients if the proper medications were available. "It is very sad, but when someone comes in with multiple-drug resistant tuberculosis today, I have nothing to give for medicine," Corona said. "How is it possible that after thousands of years, we finally know what is the best way to treat tuberculosis and to save people's lives, yet here, in Tijuana, we continue to give treatment with no hope?"

⸺ The North Florida Project

Brenda Luna steers a county van through the deep nighttime darkness of rural North Florida roads, past a dog barking fiercely, ramshackle houses teeming with people. Luna, a nurse practitioner, who is white, stops the van at the labor camps and houses where many of the African-American farmworkers who stoop in the cabbage and potato fields here live in poverty, most of them in virtual slavery to their crew chiefs. On her rounds through the neighborhoods, Luna walks up to a known crack house surrounded by a chain link fence—she's heard someone isn't feeling well there.

"Hey, does anyone want to see the doc tonight?" she calls out.

"He's already gone up there," a woman yells back.

On this trip, six men eventually pile into the van to be ferried to a large mobile medical bus parked several miles away. One has a toothache, another is bothered by an old hand injury from a potato grader. Someone smells of alcohol. It's a convivial group, full of light and friendly banter. This could be just another night out on the town.

When they reach the bus, parked outside a convenience store, an intake nurse wants to know why each man has come. And then she asks pointedly, "Have you been coughing? If so, is there any blood? Have you had fevers, night sweats? Any sudden weight loss lately? Are you more tired than usual?"

These are symptoms of tuberculosis, and the litany of questions and the primary health care provided on this bus are continuing signs of the good work that began here during the period covered by the Old Disease, New Challenge grant and that continues, fueled by an uncommon commitment and humanity.

This Putnam County-based project hoped to bring comprehensive testing, treatment, and tuberculosis education to 1,500 African-American male migrant workers and about 4,000 Hispanic seasonal fernery workers. They lived in four North Florida counties—Putnam, St. Johns, Flagler, and Volusia—in an isolated society with little access to health care. The project also set out to create a tracking and referral system that would insure that migrant workers continue to get medical care for tuberculosis when they follow the changing crops up the eastern seaboard to North Carolina, Maryland, and Delaware. This system wouldn't be needed for the seasonal workers, who lived locally and didn't travel to distant fields.

A companion project ran concurrently 400 miles south in Palm Beach, Glades, and Hendry counties, where about 30,000 migrant and seasonal farmworkers resided. But without the resources to reach a much larger farmworker population, it scaled back its goals and thus achieved more modest gains.

Nationally, the 4 million men and women who work the fields and nurseries are among the most at risk for catching tuberculosis. In 1992, when the return of the disease peaked in the country, the Centers for Disease Control and Prevention found farmworkers six times as likely to get tuberculosis as all working American adults. They live in crowded, substandard housing, tend to have poor nutrition and many health problems, face impediments to health care, and often don't receive continuity of care because they move frequently.

Mindful that local farmworkers were fitting into this pattern, the project set out to break down barriers for testing and treatment and established targets it came close to meeting. Directly observed therapy was provided for all active cases and most people with latent disease. The results were impressive: The number of people with either active disease or latent infection markedly declined over the four years of the project, according to an analysis by the University of Florida's Division of Biostatistics. This would suggest, the analysis said, that the project's mass case-finding program was effective.[10] As a result of the project, tuberculosis came under control in this population.

"We found that by testing everyone and giving directly observed therapy both to people with active and latent disease we were preventing additional cases," said Cheryll Lesneski, county health administrator and the project's principal investigator. "This isn't something you would do in just any population—you do it only in a population with a high rate of tuberculosis, which our migrants had. In high-risk groups, it's money well spent, but it's not money that's available anymore."

A large number of people had active tuberculosis—15 migrants and a child of a seasonal worker who had recently emigrated from Mexico. None had a drug-resistant form. Treatment was completed by 93.3 percent of the migrants and 100 percent for the seasonals, with the one child adhering to the therapy. This essentially met the project goal of 95 percent completion for active tuberculosis cases.

In all, 1,052 migrant farmworkers and 1,209 seasonal workers were evaluated, some many times, with 28 percent of migrants testing positive for latent infection and 23 percent of the seasonals positive. About 151 migrants received directly observed preventive therapy with 77 percent completing it, while 205 seasonals were given this treatment with 86 percent finishing it. The goal had been for 90 percent of those with latent infection to complete directly observed preventive therapy.

But numbers just scratch the surface of what was accomplished here. The people who made up the staff for this project brought health care to the farmworkers on their own terms, rather than ask them to fit into a traditional 9-to-5 system they clearly wouldn't use.

Some key ingredients made this project work: A "migrant scout" with deep connections in this community found where the men would be working each day; the project was flexible, retooling quickly to solve problems; and employees worked crazy hours to make it as convenient as possible for the farmworkers. When obstacles arose, the project's workers repeatedly seemed to scratch their heads and say, "Let's try it a better way."

"There was a lot of caring going on," said project director Laurey Gauch. "The feeling of the folks here was that this was an emergency."

The project started out with one big advantage—Putnam County had laid the groundwork early and was able to avoid startup delays. In 1992, the county had found that the number of tuberculosis cases among farmworkers was on the rise; three of them had died. Putnam County's public health unit swiftly mounted an aggressive campaign to screen as many workers as possible. Staff members and a retired physician parked their vans and station wagons at fields and worked late into the night administering PPD skin tests. At first, the often-brutal crew leaders were distrustful, balking at the intrusion and the lost work time.

Cheryll Hampton, a migrant scout, had grown up in labor camps, and her participation was crucial in winning the farmworker community over and gaining access. She had entrée into the culture and persuaded crew leaders and farmworkers of the health care emergency.

"The crew leaders were ugly about us going to the camps or fields, because they really didn't care about their workers and didn't want the crews slowed down," said Hampton, whose father and grandfather had been crew chiefs, but of a kinder stripe. "They have to know and trust you to let you do it."

The county workers pulled up to the fields at times that were most convenient to the farmworkers—whether it be during work hours or after, at dawn or late at night. Sometimes a project staff member would jump onto a tractor or start pulling potatoes to replace a farmworker who needed an extensive consultation.

The screening told grim news: 70 percent of the migrants and 20 percent of the seasonal workers tested positive for tuberculosis. The numbers reflected both new infection and longstanding infection that hadn't previously been detected. They also demonstrated that the problem was greatest with the migrants, who usually lacked the family structure and support the seasonal workers had.

With limited resources, the county workers began treating the farmworkers from their vehicles, focusing most on the migrants. They soon noticed that many of them weren't taking their pills. Some had no place to store them, and others with latent infection and no symptoms lost interest because they didn't feel ill or simply didn't want to take pills for months. The county workers concluded that they needed to find funding to do more.

That's when the county applied for and secured a grant from The Robert Wood Johnson Foundation. With the infusion of funding, Putnam County planned to expand the screening and treatment and to provide directly observed therapy for those with active or latent tuberculosis. The grant would pay for tuberculosis education for workers, health care providers, and patients, and would go toward creating an interstate tracking system to ensure continuity of care for farmworkers as they traveled.

The farmworkers were tested each year unless they had already been found to be positive and had been treated. Outreach workers met patients with active tuberculosis in the fields or at home to watch them take their medication each day. Most of those with latent disease were also observed as they swallowed pills twice a week.

Hampton's inroads into the migrant community were critical to staying on top of testing follow-up and treatment. To be sure that outreach workers could find the highly mobile patients, she visited convenience stores and other locations where workers congregated to get the latest on where crews and individuals would be that day. As she became accepted, workers and crew chiefs would tip her and other scouts off when someone wasn't well or had a cough or other possible symptoms.

"I would be out in the field or stopping by a store where a bunch of them got coffee and someone would come up to me and say so-and-so has a cough, I know it's a tuberculosis cough," Hampton said. "This one's spitting up blood. Or they'd say that guy you're looking for, he moved to such-and-such labor camp."

The arrangement did have flaws. Patients who came for consultations lacked privacy on the medical bus. The portable X-ray machine was cumbersome to move around to different locations, and processing the film in the field was a challenge. And because a Catholic health organization furnished the bus and wouldn't allow family planning on board, the project couldn't educate workers about condoms. In addition, the county discovered that many farmworkers had other serious health problems that couldn't be treated on the bus, such as HIV, hypertension, and diabetes.

The county adapted by establishing night clinics twice a week, first with a community health clinic but ultimately solely at the county Public Health Unit office in Palatka. Using a van bought with grant funds, outreach workers drove farmworkers the 15 miles to the county clinic. There they experienced a new approach to their health care. They could get skin-tested for tuberculosis, have an X-ray taken, get tested for HIV, and have other health concerns addressed by a physician. The clinic proved to be popular. Local churches and restaurants donated meals, and a closet was well stocked with items the migrants, who traveled light, needed—blankets, gloves, socks, even toilet paper. They watched videos and enjoyed the evenings so much that they were often reluctant to leave.

"We worked until 11, 12, even 1 in the morning, and in the course of an evening saw 14 to 40 patients," project director Gauch said. "This holistic approach to the whole person created trust. They were so grateful to us. I've never worked with more appreciative and hardworking people."

The same determination was directed at developing a referral system to assure continuity of care when the migrants moved north for other crops. These efforts were less fruitful, although not for lack of trying. Many meetings were held with officials and providers in North Carolina, Maryland, Delaware, New York, and other states, and communication improved and important contacts were made. With the grant funding, the North Carolina Primary Health Care Association developed an extensive migrant farmworker resource manual. Still used today, it contains CDC guidelines for care, useful medical journal articles, and phone numbers for health departments, rural health centers, and other agencies along the East Coast migrant stream to notify when a sick worker relocates.

An Interstate Migrant Medical Record was designed, too, to standardize the information that would be relayed about farmworkers with tuberculosis, but it didn't gain lasting acceptance. The county had also hoped that a computerized farmworker data base would be the backbone of a migrant referral system. However, this became bogged down among migrant health care providers, state health offices, and the project principally because of concerns about patient privacy that couldn't be resolved. Putnam County also tried a system of faxing patient information to other providers, but it was scotched when Florida adopted new patient confidentiality rules. A plan for an outreach worker to travel with the migrants to help assure continuity in treatment for active and latent infections was also abandoned. There were too few farmworkers to follow to justify the cost.

Nevertheless, Putnam County made contacts in other states that proved useful. The county would call ahead to them to give a heads-up that an infected migrant was relocating, and to relay shared medical information. The contact would often provide the same courtesy when workers were headed back to Putnam County. This informal, low-tech networking continues today.

At present, in North Florida, tuberculosis is under control among farmworkers. When the project ended, outreach was scaled way back, and mass screenings were stopped. And although the county's public health department provides directly observed therapy to anyone in the community who needs it, including farmworkers, preventive therapy is rare.

But the spirit of this project lives on. As a direct result of the project's strong performance, the county had the credibility to secure funding from St. Vincents Health Services, Inc., and from the federal Health Resource Services Administration for a more comprehensive health care service for farmworkers—the mobile medical bus. Other gains that weren't lost include the contacts with other providers and the heightened tuberculosis awareness of farmworkers and county public health staff. And because of trust built during the project, farmworkers freely board Brenda Luna's van to be seen at these clinics two days a week. They are seen for many reasons—including Pap smears, high blood pressure, diabetes, injuries, the flu, and tuberculosis. And the nurses continue to ask whether they have any tuberculosis symptoms.

"These people are just beautiful," one farmworker aboard the van says. "They always treat you like you matter. Always."

—⁓— The Baltimore and Atlanta Projects

Demonstration projects were mounted in two other locations: Baltimore and Atlanta.

A collaboration between Johns Hopkins University and a group of churches had hoped to test whether neighborhood health workers offering financial incentives could increase voluntary screening and treatment in a low-income East Baltimore neighborhood. But the project found that the city's own tuberculosis control program had been so effective that the infection rate was very low and the project actually wasn't needed. It was consequently trimmed way back. The project did demonstrate, however, that the outreach workers from the community, who were to test, refer, and counsel residents and people in high-risk settings like prisons, needed considerably more training and supervision.

The outreach workers were also to staff a health care referral system for prisoners with latent infection who were about to be released, but this never worked out. The prisoners did, however, produce a comic book, "2 B TB Free," to encourage inmates to complete their treatment after release.

Atlanta had the highest tuberculosis rate of American cities in 1991, and its project made some headway toward fostering coordination among the many groups that until then had worked separately on tuberculosis control. A broad coalition that was established included the county and state health departments, the public Grady Memorial Hospital, Emory University School of Medicine, Morehouse School of Medicine, Mercy Mobile Health Care, correctional facilities, the CDC, and the American Lung Association.

This project conducted a mass screening—7,246 people at high-risk locations—and concluded that it wasn't an effective way to bring latent tuberculosis under control. Just 20 percent of the patients completed their six-to-nine-month drug regimen. "Until it's possible to give directly observed preventive therapy or some other therapy, treatment for latent infection is doomed to fail," said Dr. Henry Blumberg, the project's principal investigator.

An attempt to increase care for patients discharged from the hospital got good results. Outreach workers, or liaisons, met with patients in the hospital to arrange care at a local clinic after release. About 58 percent of the patients had been lost to follow-up in 1992, but just 6 percent were lost after the grant's first year. And the median time from discharge to follow-up care dropped from 81 days in 1992 to just six in 1994.

The Atlanta project made progress in creating a tuberculosis computer network and a data base for reporting and confidential sharing of patient data. This system, expected to be up and running by the end of 2001, was to centralize information that had been dispersed at various locations. It will link all providers, improving communication among them, and also surveillance and control. The state of Georgia will maintain the system.

The grantee also published the "Georgia TB Reference Guide," a pocket-sized health care education handbook that was started under the grant and has been updated since with state funding. It offers treatment guidelines for latent infection and active disease based on CDC recommendations, and lists resources and phone numbers. "It's a little book physicians put in their white coat and fits in very nicely," Blumberg said.

—— Related Grants

The Robert Wood Johnson Foundation funded a number of smaller, related grants that supported tuberculosis control efforts.

One that attracted considerable notice used mathematical modeling to predict how much treatment it would take to eradicate tuberculosis worldwide. The modeling team, led by the mathematical biologist Sally Blower, currently at the University of California, Los Angeles, developed mathematical equations that described many aspects of how the tuberculosis epidemic behaves. The models, which were published in *Science* in 1996, identified the outcomes that could be expected from a range of treatment strategies for latent and active disease. The forecasts generated interest and controversy because they found that the number of patients the World Health Organization called for treating would not lead to global disease eradication.

Another grant set out to answer one of the major ethical questions of this epidemic: Just what do we do when tuberculosis patients refuse to take their medicine and endanger other people's health? Led by Bernard Lo, a team at the University of California, San Francisco, studied all 50 states' policies on criminal and civil detention and tuberculosis case reports in California counties. The study found that with sanatoria long closed and no money to pay for hospitalization, counties often had no alternative to incarcerating people. Many counties used criminal detention as a last resort, but others imposed it more aggressively. The major upshot of this grant was a collaboration with the state of California that led to civil—as opposed to criminal—confinement in two newly created state facilities for those who fail less restrictive measures. The facilities also provide some counseling, drugs, and other services.

Another grant provided support to the National Coalition to Eliminate Tuberculosis, a group of 70 organizations working to coordinate tuberculosis control. With the grant, the coalition hired a coordinator and a support staff person, improved communication among members through an online bulletin board and a newsletter, held an annual meeting and quarterly task force conference calls, and conducted tuberculosis awareness campaigns.

—— Conclusion

One aspect of the projects merits special mention. Whatever the location, staff members with an uncommon humanitarian zeal energized the projects. Workers stretched out a hand to forgotten, often ignored people, doing unseen and dedicated work. One project worker after another wouldn't accept the idea that people down on their luck and with no money were suffering and dying needlessly from a curable disease. So they rode out in the dead of night on lonely roads to find farmworkers living in ramshackle trailers. They put in long hours for relatively low pay, to be exposed to a disease that is not only highly infectious but also is sometimes resistant to drug treatment—and they did it gladly. They were an inspiring breed.

While three years is probably too short a time period for complex projects involving hard-to-reach people to plan, operate, and show definitive results, the projects demonstrated that disaffected people *can* be reached when local government, community groups, and health care facilities collaborate. But the partners must be compatible and committed to the work. Most important, health workers must be sensitive to the culture of their potential clients, and projects must be flexible and willing to change preconceived notions to meet actual circumstances. In addition, screening for tuberculosis should be targeted toward at-risk populations and must be paired with directly observed preventive therapy and directly observed therapy. Given the ease with which diseases can spread across borders, binational work is increasingly essential, yet the challenges posed by different cultures, financial circumstances, and legal structures are daunting.

Over the life of the grants, most of which were extended to a fourth year, the alarming rise in tuberculosis was stunningly reversed, and the disease again came under control. As a result of aggressive efforts to strengthen control, tuberculosis rates declined 34 percent from 1992 to 1999, when 17,531 people were diagnosed with tuberculosis.[11] The disease was at its lowest recorded level of 6.4 new cases per 100,000 people in 1999.[12] Improvement came at a high cost, however. In New York City alone, it took more than $1 billion to rebuild a public health apparatus to meet the need.[13]

There is always a danger of tuberculosis re-emerging. A report by the National Academy of Sciences' Institute of Medicine, issued in 2000, warned the United States to maintain and even step up its tuberculosis control, to be sure it doesn't repeat history. "The question now confronting the United States is whether another cycle of neglect will be allowed to begin or whether, instead, decisive action will be taken to eliminate the disease," the Institute of Medicine said. Much more headway remains to be made among foreign-born people in this country. The number of cases among those here from foreign lands has mushroomed from 24 percent of active tuberculosis patients in 1990 to 43 percent in 1999. Almost half of these patients were natives of three countries—Mexico, the Philippines, and Vietnam—and many likely came here with latent infection.[14]

"Until we can make tuberculosis go away in places like South Africa and Tijuana, people will still be able to bring it into the U.S., even if we keep working on pockets, " said Rany Condos, co-director of the Chest Service at New York's Bellevue Hospital. "That's why we need the infrastructure to remain. I hope we've learned this from the epidemic."

Notes

1. Personal communication with Ian Smith of the World Health Organization's Stop TB Program, May 17, 2001, and with Elizabeth Lancet of the American Lung Association, May 17, 2001.
2. Institute of Medicine, *Ending Neglect: The Elimination of Tuberculosis in the United States* (Washington, D.C.: Institute of Medicine, 2000), p. 21.
3. "A Strategic Plan for the Elimination of Tuberculosis in the United States," *Morbidity and Mortality Weekly Report*, 1989, April 21, volume 38, number S-3, pp. 1–25.
4. Institute of Medicine, *Ending Neglect: The Elimination of Tuberculosis in the United States* (Washington, D.C.: Institute of Medicine, 2000), pp. 21 and 35; Centers for Disease Control and Prevention, *Reported Tuberculosis in the United States, 1999* (Atlanta, Georgia: Centers for Disease Control and Prevention, 2000), p. 9.
5. Institute of Medicine, *Ending Neglect: The Elimination of Tuberculosis in the United States* (Washington, D.C.: Institute of Medicine, 2000), p. 26.
6. J. L. Stanford, J. M. Grange, and A. Pozniak, "Is Africa Lost?" *The Lancet*, 1991, volume 338, number 8766, pp. 557–558.

7. N. W. Schluger, R. Huberman, R. Holzman, et al., "Screening for Infection and Disease as a Tuberculosis Control Measure Among Indigents in New York City, 1994–1997," *International Journal of Tuberculosis and Lung Disease,* 1999, volume 3, number 4, pp. 281–286.

8. County of San Diego Department of Health Services, Public Health Services, *Statement of Work,* unpublished report to The Robert Wood Johnson Foundation, U.S.–Mexico Tuberculosis Control Model, Section C.

9. S. Duerksen, "Tuberculosis: When Disease Knows No Boundary," *San Diego Union-Tribune,* December 28, 1997, p. A-16; and personal communication with Kathleen Moser, who is in charge of San Diego County tuberculosis control and project principal investigator.

10. Department of Biostatistics, University of Florida, "Comprehensive TB Case Finding in the East Coast Migrant and Seasonal Farm Workers in Northeast and South Florida," unpublished, 1998.

11. The incidence of tuberculosis was dramatically reduced as federal, state, and county governments pumped money into strengthening control programs that identified people with the disease, chose appropriate medications for them, and made sure that they completed treatment. Key to this effort were the use of directly observed therapy to help patients stick to their long course of treatment and stepped-up control in group-living settings, such as homeless shelters, hospitals, and prisons. Institute of Medicine, *Ending Neglect: The Elimination of Tuberculosis in the United States,* (Washington, D.C.: Institute of Medicine, 2000).

12. Centers for Disease Control and Prevention, *Reported Tuberculosis in the United States, 1999* (Atlanta, Georgia: Centers for Disease Control and Prevention), p. 2.

13. Institute of Medicine, *Ending Neglect: The Elimination of Tuberculosis in the United States* (Washington, D.C.: Institute of Medicine, 2000), p. 2.

14. "Preventing and Controlling Tuberculosis Along the U.S.–Mexico Border," *Morbidity and Mortality Weekly Report,* 2001, volume 50, number RR-1, p. 4.

CHAPTER THREE

⁓ Programs to Improve the Health of Native Americans

Paul Brodeur

> *Over 100 years ago, the Indian people of this nation purchased the first pre-paid health care plan, a plan that was paid for by the cessation of millions of acres of land to the United States.*
>
> *Senator Daniel Inouye*[1]

Editors' Introduction

The 2.5 million Native Americans living in the United States face significant health problems, including high rates of infant mortality, diabetes, and alcoholism. Conquest and the resulting system of reservations characterized by poverty and hopelessness go far in explaining the compromised health of Native Americans, but many factors are at work.

Solutions to the health problems of Native Americans have been elusive. Since the 1800s, the United States government has had the obligation to provide health care services for American Indians. Before the 1950s, this obligation was characterized by extreme neglect, and worse. Even with the establishment of the Indian Health Service in 1955, resources have remained scarce.

Native American groups form sovereign nations and have their own beliefs and traditions. Programs designed to improve the health of Native Americans, if they are to be effective, must respect these beliefs and traditions and be culturally sensitive. With these precepts in mind, The Robert Wood Johnson Foundation funded two national programs to improve the health of American Indians.

In this chapter, Paul Brodeur, a veteran writer for *The New Yorker* and a frequent contributor to the *Anthology* series, examines these two programs. The first, Improving the Health of Native Americans, allowed grantees to develop projects addressing any type of health problem they chose. The second, Healthy Nations, focused on substance abuse. Both programs gave tribes and Indian organizations wide latitude in developing strategies consistent with their own values.

This degree of flexibility was unusual for the Foundation. Even so, it has not always been easy to bridge the divide between a large, modern East Coast foundation and tribal groups having their own traditional approaches. The programs have raised a number of important issues, such as: How important is it to establish measurable goals? How can programs be evaluated objectively? Given the intractable social problems, what is an appropriate time period to look for results? How can a foundation best develop capacity within the tribes so that something is left when the project ends? Are programs like these simply drops in the bucket from a distant philanthropy?

These issues have implications beyond programs to improve the health of Native Americans. Indeed, they are relevant for any program where a donor is working across cultures with groups that have different outlooks, priorities, and values.

I n a 1985 report for The Robert Wood Johnson Foundation, Dr. Emery Johnson, director of the Indian Health Service between 1969 and 1981, wrote that "the pervasive powerlessness of Indian communities and their inhabitants, the long history of governmental suppression, discrimination, poverty, geographic and cultural isolation, lack of education, and scarcity of employment are all major factors in the etiology of Indian alcoholism." Johnson's report, entitled "The Health of American Indians/Alaska Natives: Progress, Problems, and Potential," provided the background for two national programs designed to improve the health of the Native American population: Improving the Health of Native Americans, and Healthy Nations: Reducing Substance Abuse Among Native Americans.

As Johnson suggested in his report, the health of American Indians and the development of programs to improve it can be understood only in the context of their unique history of suppression and their cultural and geographical dislocation at the hands of the Europeans who settled North America. Nothing can undo such a history, of course, but thanks to an unprecedented apology that was delivered in the summer of 2000 by Kevin Gover, the director of the Department of the Interior's Bureau of Indian Affairs, the harsh mistreatment of the nation's indigenous peoples has become a matter of public and official record. In his apology, Gover said, "It must be acknowledged that the deliberate spread of disease, the decimation of the mighty buffalo herds, the use of the poison alcohol to destroy mind and body, and the cowardly killing of women and children made for tragedy on a scale so ghastly that it cannot be dismissed as merely the inevitable consequence of a clash of competing ways of life . . . The trauma of shame, fear, and anger has passed from one generation to the next, and manifests itself in the rampant alcoholism, drug abuse, and domestic violence that plague Indian country."[2]

The Health of Native Americans

The performance of the United States government in carrying out its obligations to protect the health of American Indians was marked by decades of gross neglect. By 1900, for example, the Bureau of Indian

Affairs, which assumed responsibility for the health of Native Americans from the War Department in 1849, had only 83 physicians serving on Indian reservations; the first funding set aside specifically for Indian health—a mere $40,000—did not come until a Congressional appropriation was passed in 1911. During the next 45 years, lack of adequate funding, as well as problems encountered in the recruitment and retention of physicians and other health professionals, continued to plague the Bureau of Indian Affairs.

In 1954, Congress passed a law providing for the transfer of all functions of the Secretary of the Interior relating to Indian health to the Surgeon General of the Public Health Service, or PHS. The transfer took place on July 1, 1955, when 2,500 health workers of the Bureau of Indian Affairs, together with the Bureau's 48 hospitals and 13 school infirmaries, came under the jurisdiction of the PHS's newly created Indian Health Service.[3]

Shortly after the transfer, the Indian Health Service found that "Indians of the United States today have health problems resembling in many respects those of the general population a generation ago." This was attributed to "inadequate health services, especially preventive health services, and to substandard and overcrowded housing and lack of sanitary facilities."[4] Infant mortality among Indians was almost two and a half times that of the general population.[5] Excess mortality among Indians was attributed "almost entirely to communicable diseases for which control measures are fairly well established, and to accidents, which are increasingly recognized as a public health problem." Among the diseases found to be responsible for this excess were tuberculosis, influenza, pneumonia, and gastrointestinal diseases of dysentery, gastritis, and enteritis.[6] These accounted for approximately 25 percent of Indian deaths, but only about 8 percent of non-Indian deaths.[7]

During the next 30 years, the Indian Health Service implemented infectious disease control practices on Indian reservations. Tuberculosis and diarrheal dehydration—two major problems—were contained by early case finding, health education, the deployment of public health nurses, and, most important of all, by improving sanitation, which had been especially poor on most reservations.[8] As a result of such initiatives, infant mortality decreased by 82 percent, the maternal death rate by 89 percent, mortality from tuberculosis by 96 percent, and mortality from diarrhea and dehydration by 93 percent.[9] By 1985, tuberculosis—the fourth leading cause of death among Indians between 1951 and 1953—was no longer in the top ten; nor were gastritis, enteritis, and colitis, which together had ranked number 7. Instead, chronic diseases had become far more significant. Heart disease and cancers were among the top five causes of Indian mortality, as they were in the general population.

At the same time, diseases and causes of death in which human behavior was known to play a key role were increasing steeply. Accidents, homicide, suicide, and chronic liver disease accounted for nearly one-third of Indian deaths, compared with less than 10 percent of deaths in the general population. Alcohol abuse was noted as a major factor.[10] In fact, Indian death rates specifically attributed to alcoholism—deaths due to alcohol dependence, alcohol psychosis, chronic liver disease, and cirrhosis—were found to consistently exceed the rate of all other United States races, reaching a peak of almost 10 times the all-races rate in 1971. In addition, Indian mortality from diabetes mellitis was more than double the all-races rate, and was steadily rising.[11]

⟶ The Tension Between Modern and Traditional Medicine

Tension between modern and traditional medicine has been a recurring issue in addressing the health of American Indians. Under the leadership of Dr. James Ray Shaw, the first director of the Indian Health Service, tribal health committees were set up to try to bridge the gap between modern medical practices and traditional Indian healers, who had hitherto been banned from federal facilities.[12] During the 1960s, medicine men were found to be especially important in resolving mental health problems, and programs were instituted to develop working relationships between Indian Health Service mental health practitioners and Indian healers.[13] These and other cooperative efforts continued under succeeding directors, and were a prime emphasis of Emery Johnson, the fourth director of the Indian Health Service. A passionate believer in Indian self-determination, Johnson dedicated himself to preparing the tribes to manage their own health affairs.

Johnson's efforts to gain self-determination for his Indian clients were also aided by President Richard Nixon, who, in a dramatic policy statement to Congress on July 8, 1970, ended the 1953 federal policy of tribal termination, under which tribes in selected states had been set free of all federal controls and support. Nixon's statement initiated a policy of Indian self-determination.

Early steps toward tribal control of health matters had been taken in the middle 1960s with programs financed by President Lyndon Johnson's Office of Economic Opportunity to deploy community health representatives, who were trained by the Indian Health Service in principles of health, sanitation, communication, first aid, and home nursing. The impact of the community health representatives was especially great on large, remote reservations, where, because the Indian residents lived in small and widely scattered communities, it was not feasible to send or station physicians and nurses.[14]

However, the most far-reaching step in attracting tribal involvement to resolve tribal health problems came with the passage of the Indian Health Care Improvement Act, in 1976. In this legislation, which authorized more than $1 billion to supplement the regular Indian Health Service appropriation, Congress affirmed the "Federal Government's historical and unique relationship with, and resulting responsibility to, the American Indian people." Congress also declared that a "major national goal of the United States is to provide the quantity and quality of health services which will permit the health status of Indians to be raised to the highest possible level and to encourage the maximum participation of Indians in the planning and management of those services."[15] The law stipulated that each tribe identify its own health needs and then design a comprehensive plan to meet those needs. This requirement was met by more than 90 percent of the 508 tribes that had by then been accorded tribal status by the Bureau of Indian Affairs, and were thus considered to be federally recognized tribes.[16]

The Indian Health Care Improvement Act was also designed to extend the services of the Indian Health Service to Indians living in urban areas. At the time of its passage, 1.2 million Indians were living in the United States, roughly half on reservations and half in cities—chief among them Minneapolis-St. Paul, Seattle, and San Francisco. Because these urban Indians lacked education and job training, and because they were separated from their land and families, their condition was no better than that of their kinfolk who lived on reservations. Moreover, because Indians who left their reservations were no longer considered by the government to be Indians, urban Indians had been cut off from federal services specifically designated for American Indians, including health care.[17]

—— The Robert Wood Johnson Foundation's Program to Improve the Health of American Indians and Alaskan Natives

Emery Johnson noted in his 1985 report that there were five critical health areas affecting American Indians and Alaskan natives—alcoholism, diabetes, high infant mortality, child health problems, and chronic diseases of the aged. He singled out the importance of alcohol abuse and noted that there had been many attempts—essentially undocumented—to prevent alcoholism among Indians through active intervention with Indian youth. "Examples include therapeutic recreation programs, sports, individual tutoring in schools to enhance individual self-worth, provision of active alternatives to the drinking society, and utilization of Indian culture and religion to provide a stable self-acceptance to avoid alcohol abuse," Johnson wrote. "Careful comparison of the factors involved in these attempts at prevention, identification of those which seem to be related to a successful outcome, and design of prospective studies to validate successful interventions would appear promising."[18]

Based in part on Johnson's report, The Robert Wood Johnson Foundation launched, in October, 1988, a four-year program called Improving the Health of Native Americans by inviting Indian tribes and community organizations that serve them to submit proposals designed to prevent disease and injury, and to improve health care for Indian infants, children, adolescents, and the elderly. Tribes and organizations submitting proposals were urged to focus on some of the major causes of mortality and morbidity among American Indians. The director of the Foundation's Improving the Health of Native Americans was Timothy Taylor, a member of the Kiowa Tribe, who was an assistant professor of health administration at the University of Oklahoma College of Public Health, in Oklahoma City. "What's unique about this initiative is that tribes are being given the opportunity to address their health needs from their own environment and perspective," Taylor said at the time. "The Foundation is encouraging Indian tribes to be imaginative and creative with their proposals."

During three grant award cycles between 1989 and 1991, The Robert Wood Johnson Foundation awarded $6.2 million to 36 tribes and tribal agencies to begin health projects. (At the time, there were 515 federally recognized Indian tribes—318 in the lower 48 states and

197 in Alaska—and approximately 1.5 million people who identified themselves as Indian living in the nation.) The 36 tribes and agencies receiving grants were located from Maine to California, and from Alaska to North Carolina, and the approved projects dealt with a wide range of problems:

- The Aroostook Micmac Council, Inc., of Aroostook, Maine, undertook to reduce the level of child abuse and neglect among the Micmac with a program of education designed to break down a climate of denial.

- The Blackfeet Tribe of Montana attempted to reduce the incidence of domestic abuse on the Blackfeet Reservation in the north central part of the state by implementing educational programs designed to encourage batterers to discontinue their pattern of violence.

- Central Valley Indian Health—an organization serving Indians living in the Central Valley of California—sought to reduce the incidence of substance abuse among Indian adolescents with counseling sessions, and by holding community workshops that encouraged a return to traditional tribal values.

- The Ganado Unified School District No. 20 Foundation, in the Navajo Nation of northeast Arizona, developed and implemented a comprehensive program focusing on maternal and infant care.

- The Grand Traverse Band of Ottawa and Chippewa Indians, located in northwestern Michigan, undertook to prevent substance abuse within the family (with special emphasis on children) by holding ceremonies and rituals of traditional spiritual and health practices, in order to renew selected customs and traditions of the tribe as they related to health promotion and wellness.

- The Maniilaq Association, an organization dedicated to fulfilling the health and social service needs of Native Americans living in northwest Alaska, started a project to reduce the incidence of children prenatally exposed to drugs, particularly alcohol, by seeking to empower Indian villages with the responsibility for their own health, well being, and cultural survival.

- The Minnesota Safety Council, in St. Paul, implemented a program to reduce injuries and deaths from a high incidence of motor vehicle accidents, fires, and falls among the Red Lake Band of Chippewa Indians in northern Minnesota.

- The St. Regis Mohawk Health Services, of northern New York, initiated a project to strengthen the parenting skills of young Indian mothers through mentoring, child care education, and the inclusion of mothers and grandmothers in the provision of child health care.

- The Oneida Tribe of Indians of Wisconsin sought to reduce some of the precursors of heart disease and diabetes—specifically obesity and lack of activity among youth—by developing self esteem among sixth-to-eighth graders, instituting a weight control program providing basic nutrition and starting a fitness program that emphasized traditional tribal activities.

Some projects attempted to mesh the two worlds of traditional and modern medicine. The Navajo tribe of Arizona, New Mexico, and Utah, for example, used both Navajo traditionalism and modern psychotherapy in the treatment of molested children in its project. The Navajo believe that if something evil happens to a person, he or she must have a ceremony performed in order to be rid of the evil and to restore a balance between the good and the bad. Psychotherapy alone is not considered to be sufficient to treat a sexually abused child, but must be used in conjunction with a ceremony performed by a Navajo medicine person to complete the healing process. The Navajo project also included an education program designed to prevent child sexual abuse.

In 1996, The Robert Wood Johnson Foundation awarded a grant to Lawrence R. Berger, a research scientist at the Lovelace Clinic Foundation, in Albuquerque, New Mexico, and a faculty member for the Indian Health Service's Injury Prevention Fellowship Program, to conduct a retrospective evaluation of all 36 projects that had been funded under the Improving the Health of Native Americans Program, and to prepare a monograph for Native American communities and program developers on promising models and practices. In his evaluation, which was delivered to the foundation in 1998, Berger found that Native American communities were "exploring solutions to health problems using strategies and methods rooted in their cultural, historical, and spiritual heritage." Among the culturally based approaches to improving health were the use of sweat lodges—dome-shaped structures made from mounds of earth and willow poles covered with

blankets or animal skins—which can accommodate ten or more people, who experience purification of mind, body, and spirit by sitting
in intense heat generated by pouring water over hot coals in the center of the lodge, and by singing sacred songs, telling personal stories,
and participating in rituals such as the pipe ceremony. Other culturally based activities for improving health were group counseling sessions utilizing the traditional Talking Feather; storytelling by elders;
participation in traditional crafts and singing, dancing, and drum-
ming; Indian language classes; pow-wows; discussion of historical and
spiritual issues; recreational activities such as basketry, archery, and
canoeing; and intergenerational activities with young people participating in traditional teachings and ceremonies led by elders.

Not surprisingly, Berger found that an enormous challenge to
incorporating cultural dimensions in urban programs was posed by
the fact that client populations came from different tribes and had
experienced different exposure to traditional ways. In addition, he
learned that virtually every one of the 36 projects lacked a quantitative evaluation of outcome, and that except for the perceptions of
community members, no hard data existed to demonstrate the effect
of any given program on the community's health. Among the reasons
for the paucity of evaluation data were a lack of follow-up of program
participants, the perception by some tribal members that surveys of
substance abuse were threatening, the confidential nature of traditional healing ceremonies, and the suspicion of Native American communities toward outsiders, including researchers. Berger also found a
lack of objective consulting and technical assistance to tribes in the
area of health services organization, financing, and management. He
recommended that in the future the blood alcohol levels in female
Indian injury victims be reviewed, hospital records be examined to
determine the incidence of fetal alcohol syndrome, and pre- and post-
program surveys be conducted to measure self-esteem, decision-making, and leadership skills among young people and adults who
participate in projects.[19]

In his monograph, entitled "Model Programs in Tribal Health,"
Berger reviewed ten projects that he considered to be outstanding.
One of them was the development of a community clinic and wellness center by the Coeur d'Alene Tribe, of Plummer, Idaho. The tribe's
goal was to establish a full-time clinic, known as the Benewah Medical Center, that would be tribally owned and managed and financially
self-sustaining. In order to realize this goal, the tribe made several bold

moves. Among them was the decision to serve both the Indian and non-Indian population of the area, to construct new health care facilities in phases dependent upon utilization and financial strength, to implement a financial system so that the clinic could become self-sufficient on the basis of third-party collections, to collaborate with the City of Plummer so that the Benewah Medical Center was eligible to apply for numerous outside sources of funding, and to hire a community outreach worker to help families fill out applications for assistance. With 1,500 tribal members and 10,000 other people in its service area, the Benewah Medical Center had 8,000 registered patients by 1998. In July of that year, the Coeur d'Alene Tribe opened a 43,000-square-foot Wellness Center in Plummer, which houses a day-care program, community health services, a five-lane swimming pool, a therapy pool, a "healthy heart" snack bar, an aerobics area, wet and dry saunas, racquet ball courts, a strength-training area, a running track, and a gymnasium.[20]

Another model project cited by Dr. Berger was a motor vehicle safety program undertaken by the Navajo Nation, in Window Rock, Arizona, whose vehicle-related death rate was five times as large as that of the overall United States population. In 1988, the Navajo Nation Tribal Council decided to require the use of safety belts and infant car seats for all vehicle occupants. Cooperation for the project was established between the Navajo Department of Highway Safety, the local police, and the New Mexico Traffic Safety Bureau. A Navajo medicine man delivered a blessing for the program on Navajo radio, which reaches an audience of 60,000 people. Navajo police established roadblocks, issuing citations, and explaining to drivers the importance of wearing seat belts and using car seats for their children. Within two years, adult seat belt use rose to more than 70 percent of motor vehicle occupants, and there was a 30 percent reduction in the rate of hospitalization caused by motor vehicle injuries.[21]

Still another project cited by Berger was conducted in Lawton, Oklahoma by Kenneth Coosewoon, a Kiowa/Comanche, who is both a sweat lodge leader and a certified alcohol and drug abuse counselor. Coosewoon believes that sweat lodges can play a major role in the prevention, treatment, and aftercare of Indians with alcohol and substance abuse problems. "The sweat lodge is especially useful for individuals who are fearful of participating in any type of group work," he has said. "The process is extremely non-threatening, thereby allowing the participants to display more openness and a willingness to experience the physical and purifying effect." When Coosewoon conducts the lodge for people with substance abuse problems, he provides counseling and referrals. "The lodge is not a cure-all, it's a start," he has said. "It helps you get in touch with the Creator, to find and nurture the spiritual from within yourself. There is no membership or proselytizing, just the experience of the power of prayer. Once you get your spirituality, you can go to church, Alcoholics Anonymous, or other places."

During the one-year grant period for this project, approximately 1,400 people attended the sweat lodges. Seven lodges were built to provide aftercare and follow-up services, 13 were used as alternatives to alcohol and drug use, and 5 were established in Oklahoma prisons, in which 22 percent of the inmates are Native American—nearly triple the percentage of Native Americans in the overall Oklahoma population.[22]

~~~ The Healthy Nations Program

By early autumn, 1992, funding for the Improving the Health of Native Americans program was coming to an end. At that point, having recently adopted a new goal area to reduce substance abuse and aware that a majority of grantees under the program had elected to focus on alcohol and substance abuse, The Robert Wood Johnson Foundation announced that it planned to award $13.5 million for a new initiative called Healthy Nations: Reducing Substance Abuse Among Native Americans. Because the Foundation was already helping communities across the nation address the issue of substance abuse in its Fighting Back program, it decided to tailor a special initiative to Native American communities with a conceptual model similar to that of Fighting Back—a model that supported a broad engagement of the community in understanding the nature and extent of its substance abuse problem, as well as a process that would lead to a community-wide consensus on how to attack the problem. At the same time, Healthy Nations would incorporate, as did the Improving the Health of Native Americans program, traditional Indian cultural values into its substance abuse treatment projects.

Grants to finance the new program were to be awarded in two stages. During the first phase, up to 15 tribes and communities would receive two-year awards of as much as $150,000 to plan and develop communitywide strategies to reduce the use of alcohol, tobacco, and illegal drugs. During the second phase, the projects would be eligible for financing of as much as $1 million over a four-year period to carry out the programs developed during the planning stage.

On December 17, 1993, the Foundation announced that 15 tribes and Native American organizations would receive financing for programs designed to combat alcoholism and substance abuse by addressing contributory problems, such as a deteriorating sense of cultural heritage, a lack of consistent opposition to substance abuse within individual communities, and strong peer pressure among youth to drink, smoke cigarettes, and use illegal drugs. A wide variety of approaches was taken by the grantees. For example:

- The Confederated Salish and Kootenai Tribes of the Flathead Reservation, in Montana, undertook a media campaign to fight alcohol abuse that was operated by tribal young people.

- The Eastern Band of Cherokee Indians of North Carolina arranged for families to take in individuals who had come out of substance abuse treatment programs, thus providing them with a drug- and alcohol-free environment.

- The United Indian Health Services, in Trinidad, California, held a New Year's Eve Sobriety Pow-Wow, youth camp-outs, and a traditional stick game tournament as part of its program to fight alcoholism and drug abuse.

- The White Mountain Apache Tribe, in Arizona, formed a Men's Cluster group to address risk factors in the behavior of male substance abusers and to support non-drinking lifestyles.

- The Cherokee Nation of Oklahoma held a Nativefest emphasizing the Tribe's cultural heritage and established a health program that emphasized walking and running. The program also trained 30 people to teach smoking cessation classes and sponsored community activities such as running clubs, youth/elder camps, native games, community dinners, and highway safety and wellness classes.

- The Confederated Tribes of the Colville Reservation, in Washington, organized a Community Pride Ride featuring camping and horseback riding, as well as a sobriety and healthy choices pow-wow.

- The Minneapolis American Indian Center sponsored a performance by the Dakota Plains Dancers that was attended by 800 young people, and began a comprehensive public awareness campaign to address alcohol, drug, and tobacco abuse, using radio and television announcements, billboards, videos, brochures, posters, flyers, and a quarterly newsletter.

- The Friendship House Association of American Indians, in San Francisco, sponsored a traditional youth gathering attended by 350 young people and 80 volunteers.

- The United Indian Health Services—by then based in Eureka, California—hired outreach workers to hold community events in remote townsites, some still without electricity, in order to bolster the morale of Indians living in outlying areas, who often had to deal with discrimination on the part of their white neighbors.

- The White Mountain Apache in Arizona sponsored outings to sacred sites, a media campaign using radio and videos to promote parent/child communication, and a rope and obstacle course that was navigated by 500 young people.

In late November, 2000, this writer traveled to Denver and spent two days with Timothy D. Noe, who has been deputy director of the Healthy Nations National Program Office since 1998. A large, friendly, and candid man, Noe is an expert in alcohol and drug abuse prevention, and, having visited all 15 grantees many times, is familiar with the programs operated by each of them. Early in our conversations, he pointed out that a great disparity in alcohol and substance abuse habits, as well as varying attitudes toward alcohol and substance abuse, exists from tribe to tribe. "The Southwestern tribes have one of the lowest cigarette-smoking rates in the United States, whereas the Plains Indians have one of the highest, so it wouldn't make much sense for Southwestern tribes to put a lot of resources into non-smoking campaigns," Noe said. "Moreover, some tribes have far higher drinking rates than others, so it makes sense for those tribes whose members are experiencing serious problems with alcohol addiction to place special emphasis upon dealing with alcoholism."

Noe went on to say that the drinking habits of some tribes were undoubtedly affected by the fact that certain reservations—for example, the Sioux Reservation at Pine Ridge, South Dakota—are close to towns that are filled with bars and package stores catering to Indians.

Noe noted that drug abuse continues to be a serious problem for American Indians. According to statistics released in July, 1998, by the federal Substance Abuse and Mental Health Services Administration, nearly 20 percent of Native Americans age 12 and older reported using illegal drugs, as compared to 11.9 percent for the total United States population.[23] The drug abuse problem among Indians is especially severe in urban areas with large Indian populations, such as Seattle, Minneapolis-St. Paul, and San Francisco, perhaps a reflection of the distressing poverty that characterizes the urban Indian's lot. In 1990, the per capita income for the 23,000-member American Indian population of the Minneapolis-St. Paul metropolitan area was less than half that of whites, Indian unemployment was nearly 20 percent, and more than 60 percent of Indian children lived below the poverty line. In addition, nearly 75 percent of Indian families with children were headed by a single parent, Indian high school students had a dropout rate twice that of white students, and more than 30 percent of Indian people 25 years of age and older had not completed high school.[24]

According to Noe, the Healthy Nations program has had to deal with drug abuse on a number of Indian reservations. "Not long ago, there was an epidemic of hepatitis C caused by the careless exchange of dirty needles among heroin-using members of one of the northwestern tribes," he said. "In order to combat the situation, the tribe's Healthy Nations project helped start a drug court, under which young people arrested for possession of illegal substances were not packed off to jail but were required to take part in a drug counseling program."

Following two days of discussions at the National Program Office, Noe and I flew to Tulsa, rented a car, and drove southeast about 50 miles on Highway 51 to the town of Tahlequah, headquarters for the Cherokee Nation Healthy Nations program, which serves the 65,000 Cherokee people living in the 14-county region of northeastern Oklahoma known as the Tribal Jurisdictional Area. There we visited for an hour with Lu McGraw, interim program director; June Maher, a health educator; and Ida Sue Grey, a public health educator, who described some of the projects that make up the Cherokee Healthy Nations program. Among these projects are safety and injury prevention education, a kindergarten-to-sixth-grade school health curriculum called The Great Body Shop, breast and cervical cancer education, running clubs, diabetes education, AIDS and HIV education, Indian heritage clubs, summer youth fitness camps, fetal alcohol syndrome education, smoking cessation courses, and school wellness programs that have been instituted in 21 of the 100 schools in the Tribal Jurisdictional Area. As part of the school wellness programs, a registered dietician visits each school once a month to deliver a lesson to students on how to fix healthy snacks and meals, in the hope that it will encourage their parents to do the same.

⟶ Assessing the Healthy Nations Program

From the outset, vast differences in cultural outlook and personal attitude, as well as the necessity of dealing with people living in large geographic areas, have made it difficult to apply orthodox standards in assessing the degree of success achieved by the recipients of Healthy Nations program grants. A good example of just how difficult can be found in a 1993 report written by Norman Dinges, professor of psychology and public policy at the University of Alaska, in Anchorage. The report attempted to evaluate the first two years of one tribe's Healthy Nations program, and was designed to answer questions about the nature of the alcohol and drug abuse initiative being instituted by the tribe, as well as the manner in which the goals of the initiative were being put into operation. In cooperation with the federal government and the reservation community, the tribal council had already established an alcohol abuse and prevention program that included alcoholic beverage control policies, school and community alcohol abuse and prevention education, outpatient counseling, and off-reservation inpatient alcohol abuse treatment. However, efforts to combat serious alcohol and substance abuse were fragmented, and only when the Healthy Nations program came into being were sufficient efforts made to mount a coordinated attack on the problem.

From the beginning, the Healthy Nations program functioned within the oversight of the tribal council and its chairman, the tribal health administrator, and the tribal health and welfare committee. However, issues of territoriality arose when certain individuals felt left out of the program's planning and development process, when the program was seen as a potential competitor for limited budgetary resources, and when it was seen by some people as an indirect evaluation of the quality of previous efforts to combat alcohol and substance abuse. Issues of territoriality also arose when early Healthy Nations meetings were scheduled to be held in the tribal counseling center—the location of the Healthy Nations program office—and not in the tribal treatment and aftercare facility.

In his report, Dinges praised the Healthy Nations program by declaring, "Seldom if ever have the alcohol and substance abuse problems on the reservation been approached as a multifactoral problem in which all relevant agencies are working together to understand their part in the problem and their contribution to the solution." At the same time, he expressed uneasiness over the complex pattern of resistance to change that he had found on the part of many tribal members.

In September of 1997, Dinges submitted an analysis to the National Program Office of the Healthy Nations projects undertaken by three other Indian nations. He found that extensive political changes within one tribe's health division had limited the number of tribal departments with which the Healthy Nations program could interact. He also found that as the primary facilitator of Healthy Nations links to the community, the tribal council required program coordinators to clear all advertising and press releases through its tribal public affairs office. Such constraints did not exist in the Healthy Nations programs of the other tribes.

One of the most interesting aspects of Dinges's report was his comparative analysis of group belief systems within the three grant recipients. A cardinal feature of the Healthy Nations program operated by one nation was that a coalition of people and agencies had formed a strategic alliance around the belief that their mission transcended individual aspirations. Among another, however, there was considerable disagreement over whether traditional tribal values and practices were the best way to reduce and prevent substance abuse, as well as conflicting beliefs about the problem among Healthy Nations program staff members, tribal administrators, and members of the community at large. According to Dinges, no fewer than thirty different religious sects exist among this nation, ranging from Catholics and Lutherans to traditionalists, who hold puberty ceremonies that are considered to be pagan by some members of the tribe. For its part, the third nation had to contend with a diffuse and complex set of beliefs held by people living in the region regarding the reduction and prevention of substance abuse, including a widespread belief in native vulnerability to substance abuse.

In each of the years 1998, 1999, and 2000, Dinges submitted to the National Program Office Comparative Site Reports for the Healthy Nations programs operated by five Indian nations. Dinges's findings varied widely from program to program. For example, in his report of July 30, 2000, he found that identification and assessment of substance abusers was proving to be a major challenge for the Healthy Nations staff members of one tribe, who had not been trained for the task and had to rely on other tribal programs to carry out the function. In contrast, he reported that another tribe had developed a robust early identification and assessment program, and had provided alcohol and drug abuse education classes to 700 community members. In yet another program, he learned that although restrictions on the counseling roles of staff members had been lifted, referrals to other tribal agencies, even when there were indications of physical and sexual abuse, were not always acted upon.

Like Professor Dinges, Timothy Noe believes that an orthodox evaluation of the Healthy Nations program will be difficult. In order to be sensitive to Indian sovereignty, he says, The Robert Wood Johnson Foundation designed Healthy Nations to be planned and directed from within the Indian community, with the result that no formal evaluations of the various projects were conducted while they were in progress. Recently, however, the Foundation awarded grants for formal assessment of the programs to Professor Dinges and to Philip May, professor of sociology and psychiatry, and director of the Center on Alcoholism, Substance Abuse, and Addiction, at the University of New Mexico in Albuquerque. Dinges will conduct a systematic analysis of historical attempts to deal with alcoholism and substance abuse among the grantees prior to the Healthy Nations initiative, and will look in greater detail into the varying attitudes and responses of the grantees toward the problem. Professor May will conduct a statistical analysis of a series of indicators—accident investigations, alcohol- and drug-related arrests, clinic visits, and such—to see if any trends can be observed. Their findings are expected to be ready in the autumn of 2003.

Meanwhile, Healthy Nations grantees are carrying out a range of interesting programs. The Seattle Indian Health Board under the leadership of director Steve Gallion has developed mentoring programs with the Boeing Corporation, Microsoft, and the American Indian Academy of Science and Engineering. As a result of the Microsoft program, Indian youth are better prepared to participate in the company's High School Internship Program, which provides young men and women with the skills to be employed by Microsoft. Mike Goze, director of the Minnesota American Indian Association's Healthy Nations program, has instituted a large and well-attended recreational program, and has successfully expanded the mentoring project to include non-Indian mentors. Under the leadership of Wayne Grigsby, the Healthy Nations program of the Friendship House Association of American Indians in the San Francisco Bay Area has sponsored a comprehensive sports program, a traditional youth gathering, a parenting program, an after-school drop-in program, an annual youth conference, and an annual celebration for families whose members are recovering from alcohol and substance abuse. Still another program has been operated by the United Indian Health Services, in Eureka, California. Its director, Jim McQuillen, who became a school board director in a northern California county that was notorious for discriminating against its Indian residents, managed to persuade his fellow board members to establish cultural sensitivity programs in their schools. The Eureka program also sponsors cultural awareness projects, after-school programs, youth counseling on substance abuse and appropriate sexual conduct, an Elders Conference, a Family Fun Day, Teen Advisory Groups, and efforts to curb teenage smoking.

—⁓— Conclusion

As the Healthy Nations program has drawn to a close, possible directions for future Foundation-sponsored initiatives have been suggested by the co-directors of the National Program Office—Spero Manson, a Pembina Chippewa, who is professor and head of the Division of American Indian and Alaska Native Programs of the Department of Psychiatry at the University of Colorado Health Sciences Center, in Denver, as well as director of the University's National Center for American Indian and Alaska Native Mental Health Research Center, and Candace Fleming, who is an assistant professor in the Division of American Indian and Alaska Native Programs. One of their suggestions is that the Foundation make Native American communities aware of other Foundation programs for which they might be eligible to apply by establishing an office to educate Indian tribes about such programs, and to provide them with the necessary technical assistance to write grant proposals. (One conclusion to be drawn from the analysis of the Healthy Nations program is that most Indian tribes and communities lack the experience and training to write competitive grant proposals.)

A second suggestion, building on strategies that were employed by the Healthy Nations programs of the Cherokee Nation of Oklahoma, the Minneapolis American Indian Center, Northwest New Mexico Fighting Back, Friendship House Association of American Indians, and the Cheyenne River Sioux, advocates culturally based recreational activities—such as horseback riding, lacrosse, running, dancing, and sweat lodges—as vehicles for improving the physical and emotional health of Native American communities.

Manson and Fleming also suggest building leadership capacity for planning, programming, and policy in American Indian and Alaska Native communities—something for which the Healthy Nations program has demonstrated a pressing need—and developing a mental health care initiative that would address the unique social, cultural, economic, and geographic landscape of American Indian and Alaska Native communities.

As the cost of health care has risen, the inadequacy of government appropriations for Indian health has become increasingly evident. Some experts believe that the burden now being placed on Indian tribes to provide resources to supplement government appropriations accounts in large measure for the epidemic of casino gambling that has swept through Indian country in recent years, and that if the erosion of the federal role continues, the ultimate outcome may, in effect, become termination of federally designated Indian status in the nation.[25]

Such an outcome would, of course, undo the long struggle of Native Americans to achieve true standing in their land of origin, as well as an undoing of the efforts of the Indian Health Service and of foundations such as Robert Wood Johnson to improve the health of American Indians. It would also make a mockery of Senator Inouye's poignant reminder that more than a century ago the Indian residents of the United States purchased the first pre-paid health care plan in history by ceding millions of acres of land to the United States. Indeed, it would place Native Americans, who have been the victims of neglect and discrimination, in the unfair position of having to pay an exorbitant price for their health care plan not once but twice.

Notes

1. A. B. Bergman, D. C. Grossman, A. M. Erdrich, et al., *Political History of the Indian Health Services*, The Milbank Quarterly, volume 77, number 4, 1999, p. 601.

2. Remarks of K. Gover, Assistant Secretary for Indian Affairs, Department of the Interior, at the Ceremony Acknowledging the Establishment of the Bureau of Indian Affairs, September 8, 2000. http://www.doi.gov/bia/asia/175gover.htm.

3. A. B. Bergman, D. C. Grossman, A. M. Erdrich, et al., *Political History of the Indian Health Services*, The Milbank Quarterly, volume 77, number 4, 1999, p. 577.

4. E. A. Johnson, "The Health of American Indians/Alaskan Natives: Progress, Problems, Potential," unpublished report to The Robert Wood Johnson Foundation, 1985, p. 21.

5. Ibid, p. 26.

6. Ibid, p. 21.

7. Ibid, p. 23.

8. A. B. Bergman, D. C. Grossman, A. M. Erdrich, et al., *Political History of the Indian Health Services*, The Milbank Quarterly, volume 77, number 4, 1999, p. 580.

9. Ibid, p. 573.

10. E. A. Johnson, "The Health of American Indians/Alaskan Natives: Progress, Problems, Potential," unpublished report to The Robert Wood Johnson Foundation, 1985, pp. 25–26.

11 Ibid, pp. 29–30.

12 A. B. Bergman, D. C. Grossman, A. M. Erdrich, et al., *Political History of the Indian Health Services*, The Milbank Quarterly, volume 77, number 4, 1999, p. 581.

13. E. A. Johnson, "The Health of American Indians/Alaskan Natives: Progress, Problems, Potential," unpublished report to The Robert Wood Johnson Foundation, 1985, p. 56.

14. A. B. Bergman, D. C. Grossman, A. M. Erdrich, et al., *Political History of the Indian Health Services*, The Milbank Quarterly, volume 77, number 4, 1999, pp. 585–6.

15. Ibid, p. 591.

16. Ibid, p. 587.

17. Ibid, p. 592.

18. E. A. Johnson, "The Health of American Indians/Alaskan Natives: Progress, Problems, Potential," unpublished report to The Robert Wood Johnson Foundation, 1985, pp. 67–72.

19. L. R. Berger, *Improving the Health of Native Americans Grant Program: a Retrospective Evaluation*, unpublished report to The Robert Wood Johnson Foundation, 1998.

20. L.R. Berger, *Model Programs in Tribal Health*, unpublished report to The Robert Wood Johnson Foundation, 1998, pp. 4–5.

21. Ibid, pp. 8–9.

22. Ibid, pp. 18–19.

23. S. Kasllagher, The NCADI Report, October 29, 1998.

24. J. R. Moran, *Minneapolis/St. Paul Healthy Nations Documentation Report*, unpublished report to The Robert Wood Johnson Foundation, February 15, 1995.

25. A. B. Bergman, D. C. Grossman, A. M. Erdrich, et al., *Political History of the Indian Health Services*, The Milbank Quarterly, volume 77, number 4, 1999, pp. 600–601.

CHAPTER FOUR

⟿ Service Credit Banking

Susan Dentzer

Editors' Introduction

Over the past year, far greater attention has been given to the role of volunteers in providing social services to their neighbors and members of their communities. For example, in his commencement address at the University of Notre Dame in May, 2001, President Bush said, "We must move to the third stage of combating poverty in America. Our society must enlist, equip, and empower idealistic Americans in the works of compassion that only they can provide."

Since the 1980s, The Robert Wood Johnson Foundation has been looking for ways to encourage people to volunteer their services to those in need. Faith in Action, which funds interfaith coalitions of caregivers, is the Foundation's single largest program; it was recently reauthorized for $100 million over a seven-year period. (The program was discussed in the 1998–1999 volume of The Robert Wood Johnson Foundation *Anthology*.)

The Foundation has also given priority to expanding and improving long-term care services for elderly people, particularly those who are frail. These include three programs, described by A.E. Benjamin and Rani Snyder elsewhere in this *Anthology*, to enable disabled people to select and manage their own services, and a number of programs to make long-term care insurance more readily available to seniors.

The Foundation's interest in increasing voluntarism and in improving long-term care for frail elderly people came together in the two programs examined in this chapter by Susan Dentzer, a journalist and the national health correspondent for public television's *The NewsHour*. The programs experimented with an idea called "service credit banking," in which people volunteering to provide services to needy individuals would receive chits in a paper bank that entitled them to receive services in the future if and when the need arose. The simple *quid pro quo* approach to encouraging voluntarism was the brainchild of a social activist, attorney, and economist—himself a senior citizen—who had the drive to translate an idea into action.

The programs did not work out as hoped. In her analysis, Dentzer explores whether service credit banking—as demonstrated in the projects funded by The Robert Wood Johnson Foundation—was a good idea that was badly timed or implemented or whether it was simply a flawed idea. Different observers may reach different conclusions. Whatever the conclusion reached, the service credit banking programs did offer some lessons that informed subsequent efforts of the Foundation to encourage voluntarism.

—∿∿— "A mericans form associations for the smallest undertakings," Alexis de Tocqueville wrote around 1835.[1] It's as if he foretold a scene, some 160 years later, in which a group of frail elderly women in Minnesota would band together to make baby blankets for unwed mothers. Or as if he envisioned a tableau in which healthy retirees in Colorado volunteered to give homebound seniors car rides to their doctors' appointments. Perhaps Tocqueville's comments foreshadowed the acts of Carol Hoffman, a Virginia woman disabled and largely homebound as a result of a crippling knee injury. An active volunteer in her own way, she regularly made phone calls to cheer up similarly homebound senior citizens until her death from a heart attack at age 42.

If Tocqueville were to witness all these contemporary American scenes, he might say that Americans are people who still like to tackle problems in a group—undertakings that may loom small in the great scheme of things but large in the lives of those they touch. At the same time, though, the Frenchman probably wouldn't be surprised to learn that many of the volunteers in these modern tableaux weren't entirely motivated by altruism. They were also earning modest chits that they could later cash in for similar services. As with members of today's frequent flier airline programs, these volunteers were in some cases trading work for credits that could be used to book trips, pay car insurance premiums, or even buy vitamins out of a catalog.

This, too, would have struck Tocqueville as a familiar aspect of American character. In the United States, he wrote in *Democracy in America*, "all the members of the community are independent of or indifferent to each other," so that "the cooperation of each of them can only be obtained by paying for it."[2]

A century and a half later, we can marvel at Tocqueville's grasp of these seemingly contradictory aspects of American life: the love of community alongside the pursuit of self-interest. Indeed, that very duality lay at the heart of The Robert Wood Johnson Foundation's decade-long experiment in service credit banking—systems in which volunteers provided supportive services for frail elderly people in exchange for credits entitling them to similar services, or even to goods. The Foundation organized and largely financed this experiment in two distinct phases. From 1987 to 1990, it helped to run demonstration projects at six health care organizations, including hospitals and a nursing home. Then, from 1992 to 1999, it did the same with programs at six health maintenance organizations, or HMOs.

These experiments were designed to test the notion that systems of service credits could help narrow some of the yawning gaps in long-term care. In the end, both sets of experiments were closer to being failures than successes. Of the six programs launched at HMOs, for example, only two survived beyond the end of Robert Wood Johnson Foundation funding. As of 2001, only one was still allowing volunteers to earn and bank service credits—the other having turned into a plain-vanilla volunteer program in which people helped other people just because they wanted to.

Even so, both phases of The Robert Wood Johnson Foundation's experiment—and especially the second, formally called Service Credit Banking in Managed Care—shed light on a key question: what will it take to reorient American society so that it can meet the financial, organizational, and other demands of caring for legions of people who are frail and old? This issue is significant now, and it looms even larger for the future.

As of 1995, nearly 13 million Americans reported long-term care needs.[3] According to one recent study, family and friends of those with chronic disabilities are already supplying them, gratis, with the equivalent of almost $200 billion a year in services—helping them eat, bathe, go to the toilet, shop for groceries, balance their checkbooks.[4] What's more, that sum is on top of roughly $150 billion a year that individuals, private insurance, and public programs shell out on nursing homes and home health care. With outlays of support and dollars already so large, it's anyone's guess what they will be by 2040. Demographers project that by that point there could be anywhere from 59 million to 92 million persons over 65 living in the United States (versus 35 million at present), and anywhere from 8 million to 21 million persons age 85 or older (versus 4.4 million today).[5]

One thing seems certain: there is virtually no way that formal programs—and taxpayer funding of them—will be enough to satisfy the full range of needs of tomorrow's frail elderly people. This means that a good share of those services will have to be provided informally—by families, friends, or others giving care more or less out of the goodness of their hearts. In the age of big-screen TVs, gated subdivisions, and other barriers to civil society, how can we create surrogate communities of caregivers where none really exist? How can we mobilize people so that they not only notice that the poor old lady across town can't get out of bed—but so that they actually hop in the sport utility vehicle and drive over to take out her garbage, hold her hand, rake her lawn?

Could the answer possibly lie in something as arcane and unfamiliar as service credits? Would that same SUV driver, or anybody else, for that matter, really find value in accumulating small rewards for volunteering? To understand why The Robert Wood Johnson Foundation thought the answer might conceivably be yes, we need to pay a visit to the father of the service-credit concept—a septuagenarian named Edgar Cahn.

—⁓— The Birth of Service Credit Banking

Cahn's Washington, D.C., home is cluttered with paper and stacked high with boxes. That's in large part because it's also the home of the tiny in-house think tank he founded, the Time Dollar Institute. Cahn is an attorney, an economist, and a long-time social activist—a veteran of the 1960s War on Poverty and a friend of the consumer activist Ralph Nader. Having served in the Justice Department in the '60s's under Attorney General Robert F. Kennedy, he later went on to help found the Legal Services Corporation, the government-sponsored entity that provides attorneys for disadvantaged people. As Cahn recounts in one of his books, *No More Throw-Away People,* he viewed his vocation as fighting for others and changing the world.

In a recent interview, Cahn noted that the first phase of his social activism was motivated by a classic progressive belief that "you could use rights and advocacy to get a more equitable distribution of goods and power." But in mid-career two events challenged the underpinnings of his activism and ultimately changed its course. The first event was a major heart attack that destroyed much of his coronary capacity and left him languishing for weeks in a hospital, tended to by a retinue of roughly 20 doctors, nurses, and other caretakers. "In the hospital," Cahn says, "I learned that the helper always feels good, but the helpee doesn't necessarily feel validated or affirmed. I realized that I didn't have an identity except as a recipient. You don't feel special to others when you're in need of special support and help."

The second wake-up call followed efforts to kill or scale back funding for the Legal Services Corporation in the 1980s. Cahn noticed something peculiar at congressional hearings around that time. "Not a single client family," no one who'd been helped by Legal Services, "showed up to fight for it." The lesson? "The unilateral giving of vital services doesn't alone create a constituency for a healthy society," Cahn says today. "I think we send the wrong message inadvertently when we help people."

The result was Cahn's conversion to what was almost a neoconservative perspective—closer to the insight of a welfare reformer than to that of the Naderite redistributionist Cahn had once been. He needed an idea to link together several realities: that there were lots of people in the world who needed help. That helping them could in some ways disempower them. That to keep them feeling empowered and engaged, he needed to enlist them in helping themselves. That conventional voluntarism didn't always motivate people, because it didn't always reward volunteer work for what it was—real work. "The solution, when I hit upon it, seemed obvious," Cahn writes. "Why not bank time spent helping others—something like a blood bank? Help somebody. Give an hour, get an hour. One hour equals one service credit."

Cahn thought then, as he still believes now, that the idea would be especially applicable to elderly people. If a group of comparatively healthy elderly people could earn service credits for helping others worse off than themselves, the world would be better in several respects. Elderly helpers would not feel like useless throwaways, having been rewarded for their volunteer work through service credits. Meanwhile, the "helpees" would get the service they needed, whether it was a ride to a doctor or a lifeline against loneliness. And finally, even these helpees would know that they, too, had the option of performing at least some services for others, however minimal, much as the housebound and seriously ill woman in Virginia made phone calls to cheer up others. In the process, they, too, could earn credits and escape the debilitating downward spiral of dependency, or the sense of being a throwaway person. Helper and helpee would be connected by a sense of reciprocity: "I need what you can do in the world as badly as you need what I can do for you."

At the suggestion of his friend Nader, who thought the "service credit" terminology too clunky, Cahn eventually came up with an alternative phrase: time dollars. Today, he helps to promulgate interest in the concept and support dozens of time dollar projects around the world. One that he helped set up in Florida came to the attention of Rolando Thorne, a program officer at The Robert Wood Johnson

Foundation, who in turn brought the idea to his boss Jeffrey Merrill, who was then a vice-president at the Foundation.

The Foundation had been looking for ways to support and broaden informal assistance to seniors—a quest that, among other things, would some years later lead it to authorize up to $100 million on a separate program called Faith in Action to help churches, synagogues, and other faith institutions support their own members who needed long-term care. The notion of service credits seemed appealing in several respects, Merrill recalled in an interview. First was the idea of "getting services to people—a plumber coming in to put rails up in your bathtub, or a carpenter to secure your carpets so you wouldn't fall." Second, and "even more intriguing," Merrill said, was the notion that elderly people themselves could provide services—and that as a result, "this was a way to make them feel useful, and give them more meaning in life." And, third, "we were just floundering around for alternative financing mechanisms" for long-term care. In that context, service credits were "sort of a catchy idea."

—— The Service Credit Banking for the Elderly Program

Sensing that service credits could play a role, The Robert Wood Johnson Foundation board eventually approved the two phases of the program. The first phase, Service Credit Banking for the Elderly, authorized $1.2 million in grants for demonstration projects at six health care organizations: two hospitals, one nursing home, a senior center, a community service center, and a social health maintenance organization, or social HMO. During the program's run, from 1987 to 1990, Cahn served as an adviser. According to Robert Wood Johnson Foundation documents, the project was designed to answer three questions: would a program of service credits attract senior volunteers to serve elderly people? Precisely how important were credits themselves in this process? And could the concept increase local capacity to provide supportive services to frail elderly people?

At the end of three years, the answers to these three questions were, in effect, "Yes," "Not sure," and "Maybe." These conclusions were reached by Judith Feder, Julia Howard, and William Scanlon, three health policy experts affiliated at the time with the Center for Health Policy Studies at Georgetown University School of Medicine in Washington, D.C., who evaluated the program. They found that the programs had been effective in attracting people who were volunteering for the first time—not just "stealing" volunteers away from other programs. What's more, the programs had also accomplished a key objective in attracting elderly people to help others their own age.[6]

The evaluators spent a great deal of time and energy wrestling with how intrinsic the service credit concept had been to the success of these volunteer programs. The evidence, they concluded, was mixed. If anything, the weight of it suggested that the service credits weren't crucial either for attracting volunteers or for keeping them in the program. For example, in a survey that the evaluators conducted, only 13 percent of the volunteers said they were participating in the program to earn credits. By contrast, 64 percent said they were participating "to help others."

In the language of social science, the evaluators eventually wrote in the *Journal of Aging and Social Policy* that service credit banking organizations were "better understood as community membership organizations than as mechanical exchanges."[7] In plain English, they were even blunter. "We thought there was a lot of confusion about the value of the credits," Judith Feder recalled in a 2000 interview. The credits' role as a medium of exchange seemed overblown; if people really needed some incentive to help others, the evaluators concluded, good old-fashioned money would probably work even better. At best, they believed, the credits were little more than a tool to promote voluntarism—and in some instances, not all that effective a tool, either.

What's more, the evaluators had also discovered that in many cases the service credit banking programs weren't doing an especially good job of service credit banking—that is, of keeping track of credits as volunteers accumulated them, or of debiting volunteers' accounts when they cashed them in. "The more you thought of these programs as real banks, the less sense it made," Feder said.

Feder and the other evaluators noted other difficulties with the service credit banking organizations as well. The programs had trouble recruiting both volunteers and service recipients. They encountered a mismatch between the services older people wanted, like transportation, and the ones that volunteers were willing and able to provide. A sizeable staff was needed to recruit and manage volunteers, maintain their enthusiasm, keep tabs on those who needed services, and run the computer hardware and software that was designed to keep the whole system functioning. Moreover, because the programs didn't generate revenues and usually weren't a core piece of the sponsors' organizational missions, they were viewed as expendable, especially when difficult financial times hit. In fact, within several years after the project ended, only two of the original service credit banking programs for elderly people had survived in something close to their original form.

All that might have been enough to cause The Robert Wood Johnson Foundation to throw in the towel on the service credit concept. But the problem was this: even if service credits didn't flourish everywhere, there were at least a handful of places where the programs built around them did survive and prosper. What's more, the success of such programs was often quite impressive, and it was clear that they were delivering important services to frail elderly people that weren't being delivered elsewhere. A case in point was one of the original Service Credit Banking for the Elderly grantees, Elderplan.

Based in Brooklyn, New York, Elderplan was one of the original social HMO demonstration projects created by the federal government in the 1980s. The concept behind social HMOs was to help frail elderly people stay out of nursing homes; to achieve this, social HMOs were given waivers from the traditional Medicare and Medicaid programs, in return for which they would offer supplemental services beyond the normal benefits that these programs typically offered. The concept provided a kind of natural home for a service credit program, in that social HMOs tended to attract both enrollees and staff members attuned to the importance of providing more than just standard medical services to the aged.

At the time The Robert Wood Johnson Foundation put out its call for service-credit proposals in 1987, Dr. Dennis Kodner was the chief operating officer of Metropolitan Health System, the nonprofit health system that was the parent company of Elderplan. He knew Edgar Cahn, was already a service credit or "time dollar" enthusiast, and directed his staff to apply for a grant. Soon after, an energetic young woman named Mashi Blech joined the plan as its first and (to date) only director of the service credit program, Member to Member. As of 2001, the program was still going strong, having delivered more than 120,000 hours of services to 6,000 people over the intervening 14 years.

Just recounting these statistics, however, fails to capture the degree to which the service credit banking program at Elderplan made a difference—both in the lives of enrollees, as well as in the survival of the broader social HMO wrapped around it. As Blech described it in a 2001 interview, many of the frail elderly people already enrolled in the

Elderplan were being visited in their homes by personal care workers, who would offer assistance with such activities as bathing and toileting. Member to Member volunteers were able to augment these services with others that the personal-care workers weren't authorized or paid to perform, such as shopping or getting a ride to the doctor. That fact alone ultimately became a selling point that helped draw enrollees to the 8,000-member social HMO, said Blech. "With all the negative publicity that managed care companies get these days, Elderplan's marketing department is able to say, we're different. What other health plan would fix your leaky faucet?"

Far more than just a service organization, however, Member to Member became a living testament to the power of community-building. Members referred to the people they served as "partners," not as clients or cases, and the tales of the nearly heroic deeds some have performed testify to the caring attachments formed. Blech told of members who walked two miles through two feet of snow to make sure a "partner" had food in the house. Another—a 91-year-old woman deaf and mute since birth—was living a life of isolation and unsanitary conditions in her own home until she became the partner of volunteer Anna Colarusso. After Colarusso won the woman's trust, she virtually transformed her life—in part by persuading her to allow personal care workers into her home to provide her with needed services.

Over the years, the Elderplan time bank expanded into a range of other activities as well. Volunteers were trained as peer counselors and certified to provide education and self-help techniques for managing Alzheimer's disease, arthritis, and other conditions. As of 2001, one member, Rosalie DiPietro, was regularly leading an early-morning walking club for older people at a Brooklyn shopping mall. Others of the 200 active volunteers were engaged in activities such as conducting exercise classes by phone—calling as many as 15 other plan members at a time and coaching them through a preset exercise routine.

As Member to Member volunteers accumulated credits, Blech and her staff assembled an array of services and benefits into a package called "Credit Shop." Members could redeem credits from the catalogue for luncheons Elderplan sponsored throughout the area; bus trips for a day at the casinos in Atlantic City, New Jersey; movie theater tickets, or even a range of health-related products such as blood pressure monitors. What's more, for a number of years, members could use time dollars to defray part of the monthly premium for Elderplan until it eliminated the premium altogether in 1995.

By 2001, as Elderplan expanded its service area beyond Brooklyn and into the neighboring New York City boroughs of Staten Island and Queens, the reach of the Member to Member program grew along with it. "Our leadership had the vision and appreciation of what we had accomplished and decided to fund us fully and allow us to expand," Blech said. That sense of commitment from Elderplan's top administrators was an ingredient in other successful time dollar experiments. The top-level support of service credit banking at Elderplan was pronounced enough to provide a clue to Robert Wood Johnson Foundation officials as to what such other organizations would need to survive.

⌇ The Service Credit Banking in Managed Care Program

As the Service Credit Banking for the Elderly program wound down in the early 1990s, officials at the Foundation decided to take another tack. They believed that service credit banking organizations could be made stronger and more effective if created in an environment naturally disposed to give them institutional support and sustainability. That's when Nancy Barrand, then a Foundation program officer (and now a senior program officer), began to think about building on the experience of Elderplan—and conceived the notion of housing service credit programs in traditional HMOs around the country.

The moment seemed propitious. At that time, in the early 1990s, managed care seemed like the wave of the future in health care. Enrollment of Medicare beneficiaries in managed care organizations was growing rapidly, approaching 1.7 million in health plans nationwide. Barrand and other Foundation officials believed that managed care organizations might have the financial incentive to make service credit banking work, since supportive services that helped keep elderly people healthy and independent would probably also help to hold down costs. They also thought managed care organizations had the managerial depth and information management capabilities to keep service credit programs up and running.

In 1992, the Foundation set up a national program office for what would become the second phase of its experiment—the Service Credit Banking in Managed Care Program. As with the earlier phase, the program office was housed at the University of Maryland Center on Aging in College Park, Maryland. The director was Mark Meiners, an economist and long-term care specialist.

A search quickly began for a managed care organization that could serve as a pilot site. The first candidate was the Family Medical Group, a primary medical-care group practice in San Fernando Valley, California, that had contracts with three local HMOs. But at about the same time, Family Medical Group became the target of complaints that it was delivering inadequate care to patients. In an episode that foreshadowed later volatility at other managed care organizations, Family Medical Group lost a large HMO contract and half of its patient base, was sold to a medical management organization, and discontinued the service credit banking project.

The resulting quest for still another pilot site led to a Colorado HMO. The Rocky Mountain Health Maintenance Organization, based in Grand Junction, Colorado, was a nonprofit HMO with a commitment to serving its members, who numbered roughly 55,000 in 1993. About 8,500 of those members were 65 or older and very much in need of the types of support that service credit banking could provide. More important, Meiners says, the HMO was run by "people who wanted to make something happen."

⁓ The Pilot Program at Rocky Mountain HMO

There is an old joke about HMOs that says they have gone from being a Communist plot to a capitalist conspiracy in just two decades. In a tongue-in-cheek way, the line captures the remarkable transformation that took place as an essentially social movement within health care morphed into the multibillion-dollar managed care industry. Back when the social movement took off in the 1970s, many of the pioneers who founded HMOs did so out of a belief that they were all about preventing and treating illness, not just about cutting costs. Many saw their organizations not so much in terms of dollars and cents as in terms of building healthy communities. One HMO of this sort was Rocky Mountain. It was a place where seven-figure executive salaries were verboten—and where the original chief executive officer, Mike Weber, came on board in 1974 and was still at the helm more than 25 years later. As such, it was fertile ground when the seed of service credit banking eventually fell into it.

That happened almost by accident one day in the early 1990s. Art Crumbaker, now in his 70s, was a Grand Junction, Colorado, internist who had been one of the founders of Rocky Mountain HMO in 1972. His wife, Lucy, had read an article about service credit banking in a magazine that mentioned the earlier Robert Wood Johnson Foundation–funded experiment. She passed it along to her husband, who was interested. "I had a big geriatric practice, and I could see that there were a lot of people who could use help," he said later—whether it was getting assistance in going to the grocery store or having a volunteer handyman come in to build a wheelchair access ramp. Crumbaker thought a service credit banking arrangement would complement the Rocky Mountain HMO's other activities, and mentioned it to Weber.

Weber immediately agreed. "What struck me was that this was a logical extension of filling the needs of that [elderly] population," he recalled in an interview. The concept also fit in well with the mission of Rocky Mountain HMO. "The philosophy of Rocky Mountain had always been to try to do what's right for a particular patient," even if it went beyond providing services not traditionally thought of as health care benefits. Moreover, Grand Junction itself, situated on Colorado's Western Slope and surrounded by mountains, was a city whose geography seemed to reinforce its strong sense of community. A culture of voluntarism was already thriving: for example, a prominent local businessman and friend of Crumbaker's, Art Moss, had helped to set up a senior day care center at a local church along with other voluntary services for older people.

Weber and others got in touch with Mark Meiners, and in 1993 a three-year contract was signed to develop a time bank. The Robert Wood Johnson Foundation and Rocky Mountain HMO would each contribute $50,000 a year to the project for the first three years. The program would be housed within Rocky Mountain HMO's home health care agency, and would work, where possible, to provide services for the agency's clients. Although volunteers didn't need to belong to the HMO, only HMO members would receive services. This structure and limitations on who would obtain services was considered a temporary necessity in order to get the program up and running. The larger, long-term goal shared by Weber, Crumbaker, and Meiners was to take the time bank "into the community," as they repeatedly described it. In other words, they wished to move it ultimately beyond the walls of Rocky Mountain HMO, so that the time bank would include all of Grand Junction, drawing volunteers and service recipients alike from surrounding Mesa County and serving the entire community's needs.

The HMO set about laying the groundwork for operations and recruiting a time bank director, who arrived in 1993. Diane Dickey, previously employed at a local hospital, seemed to be the sort of enthusiastic and determined powerhouse Rocky Mountain HMO officials thought was needed to make the program fly. Their judgment proved correct. Dickey immediately began recruiting volunteers, visiting local service clubs and church groups, going "anywhere anyone would invite me," she recalled in an interview.

One of the first places she visited was the Hilltop Rehabilitation Center in Grand Junction, which held a monthly luncheon for senior citizens in the community. In attendance that day was Ted Rodda, who had just retired as an engineer for Hamilton Sundstrand Aerospace in Grand Junction, and his wife, Rita. They were interested in Dickey's description of the time bank, and decided to sign on. After a few training sessions, they were in business as two of the time bank's first volunteers.

The Roddas were not members of Rocky Mountain HMO, and so were under no illusion that they would ever be able to cash in credits to receive services. Rather, they recalled in an interview, they had a simple motivation: they wanted to help people. Ted Rodda, in particular, felt strongly about helping elderly people stay in their own homes as long as possible. "I just get a warm fuzzy feeling out of it," recalled Ted, who was born in 1927.

One of the people who became a beneficiary of the Roddas' altruism was a woman in her 80s named Bernice Burnhart, a widow whose husband had died 15 years earlier. She was legally blind and had to use a walker. "Nothing had been done to her yard for 15 years," Ted Rodda recalled, so he busied himself with her yardwork and such tasks as cleaning out the freezer. Rita helped Burnhart keep her financial affairs in order and also did the grocery shopping. As was often the case in service credit banking programs, an initial "date" between volunteer and recipient turned into a kind of a marriage. The Roddas continued to do volunteer work for Burnhart for the next two years, until her death in 1995. Clearly, a bond of friendship had developed alongside the giving and receiving of services. Says Ted, simply, "It was just a good fit. Everything seemed to go well."

As of 2001, some 8 years later, the Roddas were still volunteering for the time bank, and said in an interview that they didn't intend to give it up anytime soon. In that respect, they were typical of most of the volunteers in the program, since most stayed on for years with very little turnover. "We used to say people died to get out of the time bank," recalled Marie Schmalz, who succeeded Diane Dickey as director of the program when Dickey left Grand Junction for several years in the mid-1990s. Over the years, the volunteer ranks swelled. The local Rotary Club wanted to volunteer as a group, so they were commissioned to do yardwork. Some Rocky Mountain HMO staff members became volunteers, including Dr. Mary Clark, who also served as the time bank's medical adviser within Rocky Mountain HMO. "I pulled weeds for a lady with a breathing problem who had had a beautiful garden that had gone to waste," she said in an interview. "It made her so happy. She didn't want anything else—just wanted her garden restored."

The time bank also began to fulfill its intended function as a bank, in which people could volunteer and accumulate credits that they hoped to use later. Some senior citizens, for example, signed up to earn credits so that their spouses might be able to cash them in if they needed them someday. Among the first to both bank and draw down credits was actually a younger woman, Kathy Ireland, a Grand Junction schoolteacher in her early 30s. A single mother with two small children, she had volunteered for the time bank just a few times but then broke her leg in a car accident. Desperate for some household help, "she called up half hysterical and said, 'I only have four or five credits to cash in and I'm going to need a lot,'" Diane Dickey recalled. The time bank director told her she could receive an "advance" on her credits in anticipation that she'd earn more as a volunteer later. Dickey paired Ireland up with volunteers who pitched in with household chores and errands until Ireland recovered.

Because the time bank was set up within the home health department of Rocky Mountain HMO, as many as half of its referrals came from individuals who were receiving home health services, such as nursing visits, bathing, feeding, and other personal care. These people usually had other needs that simply weren't or couldn't be met by home health providers—for example, because particular services weren't covered by Medicare or Medicaid. This was where the services that could be performed free by time bank volunteers proved to be a godsend, said Donna Vogel, a medical social worker with Rocky Mountain HMO's home health agency. "No other group would do something like fix a broken light switch," Vogel said, noting that the cost of hiring an electrician to do that could easily exhaust a senior's monthly budget for medications. Other volunteers built wheelchair ramps or filled out applications so people could obtain free medications through special assistance programs run by pharmaceutical companies.

Perhaps the biggest unmet need for frail seniors was transportation—to get to doctors' appointments, go grocery shopping, visit relatives in nursing homes. This was especially true in Grand Junction and vicinity, which until the late 1990s had no public transportation whatsoever. As a result, anywhere from half to three-quarters of the people who drew services from the time bank got them in the form of transportation—with volunteers shuttling them to their destinations, then waiting patiently to the end of a doctor's appointment or other engagement to take them back home. Some also took the people they were providing services to on long-distance trips at their own expense, just to give them a chance to get away.

To hear those involved with the time bank tell it, the program clearly succeeded in establishing and reinforcing the sense of community that Edgar Cahn had envisioned. At annual Christmas lunches and springtime picnics, volunteers were praised for their good works by Rocky Mountain HMO officials like Mike Weber. "I surely don't live for it," said Ted Rodda, "but it is nice to hear somebody say, 'You volunteers logged 4,000 hours last year.'" At one memorable picnic, Marie Schmalz recalled, one group of volunteers was honored with special certificates; they were "retiring" from the program because they were so ill they could no longer physically perform any services. At the same event, a woman who had been receiving services from time bank while fighting breast cancer, and on Medicaid, spoke about what the program had meant to her. The woman, Jean Kissel, had eventually recovered from the cancer, gone off Medicaid, and begun working again. As she expressed her gratitude for the time bank's help that day at the picnic, "She was crying and everyone else was crying," Marie Schmalz said. The human connections Edgar Cahn had sought had been forged, and they ran deep.

The program had also succeeded in bringing to life Cahn's vision of reciprocity. For example, people drawing services from the time bank were assured that, if they chose to, they could themselves volunteer to earn credits—a fact welcomed by seniors who seemed to feel guilty and over-dependent as a result of receiving assistance. That "helped to overcome the Depression-era mentality" many of the elderly people felt, said Donna Vogel—a mentality she describes as

"I'm not going to pay someone to fix meals for me; I'll starve first." She described one homebound elderly woman, now deceased, who was for several years drawing services from the time bank but who also made regular phone calls to cheer up similarly situated seniors as a volunteer. Actions like these "made the recipient feel like they were giving back," Dickey recalled. "After a while, it wasn't always clear who was helping whom."

For all these personal successes, the program encountered serious difficulties. Running the Rocky Mountain HMO time bank was far from being a picnic. Diane Dickey and later, Marie Schmalz constantly struggled to reach a balance between the number of volunteers and the number of those who needed services. The goal was never achieved, and the latter usually outnumbered the former by around six to one. The time bank staff also labored largely in vain to get Rocky Mountain HMO physicians to refer patients to the program. Dickey reported meeting several times with the Mesa County Individual Practice Association, the doctors' group—at one point even handing out classic doctors' prescription pads imprinted with the time bank's name and phone number in the hope of jogging doctors' memories. "They were just so busy concentrating on the medical aspects of disease that they forget that when someone's discharged from the hospital, they won't be able to get their groceries," Dickey said. The result was that the time bank's services were never fully integrated into the spectrum of medical and social needs in the community.

Finally, although the time bank staff members felt strong personal and emotional support within Rocky Mountain HMO, they were consigned to working on a shoestring budget that, excluding salaries, was only about $50,000 a year. "My personal opinion is that we could have used a lot more monetary support to make the program more successful," Marie Schmalz said. In the end, the time bank was at least partly hampered by financial difficulties that faced Rocky Mountain HMO along with most managed care organizations in the latter half of the 1990s. Those strains made it impossible ever to consider expanding the program's budget, which in turn might have made it easier to enlist the aid of physicians or recruit more volunteers. As it turned out, the numbers of volunteers and people receiving services grew very little in its last few years of operation under Rocky Mountain HMO's auspices.

Eventually, these budget limits played a role in nudging the no-longer-fledgling time bank out of the Rocky Mountain HMO nest.

That, of course, had been the longstanding dream of people like Mark Meiners, Mike Weber, and Art Crumbaker—and as The Robert Wood Johnson Foundation grant period neared its end in 1998, planning began in earnest about how best to reach the goal. Several organizations in the community were approached to serve as sponsors, but for various reasons they didn't seem right. Finally, the time bank officials began talking to the Mesa County Department of Human Services, which was receptive to the idea of taking the time bank under its wing. "They said, 'We've needed this thing for so long,'" recalled Diane Dickey, who by this time had returned to Grand Junction and taken another post with Rocky Mountain HMO. County officials immediately saw the possibility of marrying the volunteer program to other services that local government was already providing to Medicaid recipients, homebound seniors, and others in need. In September of 2000, the transfer took place. The time bank moved into the Department of Human Services' offices on the outskirts of Grand Junction, while Rocky Mountain HMO agreed to contribute $7,000 annually toward the time bank's budget for at least three more years.

As of the transfer, the time bank came under the leadership of a new director, Brenda Nelson, who among other things formerly ran a food bank and worked as a Girl Scout program administrator. She evidently inherited the fervor and commitment of her predecessors, Dickey and Schmalz. In an interview, she waxed enthusiastic about her plans to "take the time bank to its next level"—that is, to broaden the pool of people it serves, as well as the services and goods that could be claimed with credits. Nelson expressed the hope that the program could double in size through recruitment of new volunteers—especially middle-aged people with older parents, who might wish to accumulate credits that could be cashed in on their parents' behalf later. She hoped to encourage major corporations to give their employees time off to volunteer with the time bank. She also planned to allow participants in six other volunteer programs run by the county to accumulate time bank credits.

Nelson's most ambitious plans centered on expanding the types of services that volunteers could claim with the credits they accumulated. She pointed to another time bank in Durango, Colorado, where volunteers who earned 200 hours of service credits can cash in 20 of them for $1 apiece to help pay car insurance or child-care bills. She wondered why volunteers in Grand Junction couldn't have similar opportunities. Or how about a catalog like the one at Elderplan in New York, where volunteers could sort through products that could be obtained with service credits, from vitamins to other health-related goods?

Nelson's enthusiasm had helped to soften an inevitable sense of let-down that some volunteers—and even Rocky Mountain HMO staff—felt when the program was transferred to the county. Volunteers from the old program were encouraged to transfer their credits to the new one, and some 80 out of 125 did so. But others, demoralized and fearful of change, dropped out; some took the attitude that "I don't want to be involved in anything with the government," Diane Dickey recalled. But others were hanging in—motivated, it appeared, by the same sense of finding meaning in their efforts to help fellow human beings. Nelson recounted the story of telling one regular volunteer that she feared she'd been calling on him too much to assist other seniors. "Don't ever think that," the man replied. "Since I lost my wife, this is what's kept me going."

—— Expanding the Service Credit Banking in HMOs Program

As the Rocky Mountain HMO pilot project picked up steam, in October, 1994, The Robert Wood Johnson Foundation authorized $750,000 for projects to replicate the time bank experiment at managed care organizations elsewhere. The goals were ambitious: the National Program Office was seeking organizations willing to attract anywhere from 500 to 1,000 volunteer caregivers over the five-year grant period. The initial response was enthusiastic, and the office received 118 requests for applications. However, about half the organizations that expressed interest didn't meet various other eligibility criteria. Ultimately, the National Program Office received only 10 completed applications by the June 30, 1995, deadline.

Five sites were eventually selected: Sentara Life Care Corporation in Norfolk, Virginia; Oxford Health Plans in Norwalk, Connecticut; CareAmerica Health Plans (now Blue Shield of California) in Woodland Hills, California; Washington State's Group Health Cooperative of Puget Sound; and Medica in Minneapolis. "We really had quite a good set of plans that stepped up to do this," said national program director Mark Meiners in an interview. But unbeknownst to the nation's most prominent health care experts, even the best managed care plans would have trouble surviving the troubles that lay ahead.

When the history of managed care is finally written, the latter half of the 1990s may go down as the era when everything went wrong all at once. Many managed care organizations that seemed to be on top of the world in the early 1990s came crashing down to earth as the decade neared its end. A case in point was Oxford Health Plans, one of the sites selected for a service credit banking project. Based in Norwalk, Connecticut, and founded by a one-time wunderkind named Stephen Wiggins in the late 1980s, by the mid-1990s Oxford had become the fastest growing HMO in America. Then Murphy's Law hit. Oxford's stock, once a darling of investors, skidded from around $70 to just a few dollars a share in a matter of weeks. The company began bailing out of its core businesses left and right, including many of its Medicare HMO plans in various states. Wiggins was ultimately fired by Oxford's board, but not before he walked away with a $9 million severance payment.

In an environment like that, it's little wonder that tiny volunteer programs like service credit banking failed to prosper. And that is exactly what happened at most of the other HMOs that wound up with service credit banking grants. Almost all these HMOs lapsed into turmoil, and were ultimately unwilling to sustain the service credit banking programs financially. For example, two of the managed care organizations, CareAmerica and Group Health of Puget Sound, either were merged or were significantly restructured during the grant period. Along with Oxford, Medica and Sentara scaled back or folded their Medicare managed care programs and shut down their service credit banking programs soon after. At Oxford, employees of the in-house service credit program showed up one day for work only to learn abruptly that much of the company's Medicare HMO business was being terminated—and as a result, the very base of their operation along with it.

Ultimately, only two of the service credit banking projects—Rocky Mountain HMO's and CareAmerica's—survived in any form whatsoever beyond the grant period. But neither of the HMOs that supported the two surviving projects were immune from the financial pressures afflicting managed care; Rocky Mountain in particular had encountered its share of red ink. The fact that the time bank survived there until 2000, while comparable programs at other HMOs didn't even make it that long, suggests that more than just the financial woes of HMOs was responsible for their downfall. In fact, the evidence suggests that commitment from senior management, and recognition that service credit banking was a valuable adjunct to the organization, were instrumental in keeping the surviving programs alive. When these were missing, the experiment was doomed to failure.

A case in point was the Sentara Volunteer Caregiving program, as the service credit banking experiment was called at the Sentara Life-Care Corporation. Sentara was a broad-based health system of hospitals, nursing homes, and physicians that also had an HMO with Medicare enrollees. After Sentara received the service credit banking grant, it recruited Leigh Hammer, the director of a local assisted living facility, to come over and run the service credit program. Housed within Sentara's LifeCare division, which operated the nursing homes and other eldercare activities, the program opened for business under Hammer's leadership in September of 1996.

Every bit as enthusiastic as her peers at the other service credit banking programs, Hammer set about the tough job of recruiting volunteers and devising a service-delivery program. It was a long, slow haul, she recalled in an interview. At the program's peak, it had a staff of no more than 160 volunteers, and served, by Hammer's estimate, just 235 people. That put it well short of the numerical goals The Robert Wood Johnson Foundation had set earlier for all the service credit banking programs. Even so, the program had developed some innovative services. Together with Sentara's home health department, Hammer helped fashion a program in which volunteers made follow-up telephone calls to children with asthma. The volunteers would conduct a telephone survey, asking whether the children were using their medications, whether they had had attacks that had necessitated visits to the emergency room, and other questions designed to ferret out whether the children were participating fully in their care. If problems were identified, a home health nurse would be dispatched to the child's home.

Although this "telephone reassurance" program was small in scale, Hammer estimated that it saved the HMO more than $100,000 just in averting unnecessary visits by home health nurses to gather similar information. Despite those savings, when push came to shove, Sentara was unwilling to invest further in the program—mainly, it seems, for lack of interest. "We made a presentation to [Sentara HMO officials] about what we were doing, and they said, 'That's real good, you take care of that over there'," Hammer recalled. "We were at a point where we needed to hire a second person, but there was no money to hire anybody else, so we couldn't grow." As a result, once The Robert

Wood Johnson Foundation grant ended, in December of 1998, so did any commitment to keeping the service credit banking program up and running. Soon thereafter, Sentara's financially troubled HMO was closed down as well.

All along, Hammer was encountering additional problems that plagued the other service credit banking sites as well. Perhaps the most frustrating was working with special computer software that had been designed for the program. The software had two basic functions: to help match volunteers with persons needing services and to keep track of the accumulating service credits. The Foundation had commissioned various software firms to develop successive generations of the software to keep pace with the change in personal computer operating systems. But almost all the versions of the software turned out to be difficult to use if not seriously flawed—even after The Robert Wood Johnson Foundation invested nearly $42,000 in a final version. "The software was pretty useless," Hammer said.

Like most of the other program administrators, Hammer ended up doing most of the matching of volunteers and those needing services in her head, or with the help of records kept in a notebook. In a sense, such small-scale actions were only symbolic of much of what happened in the rest of the service credit banking program, as once lofty expectations settled down closer to the earth.

⏤ Looking Back on Service Credit Banking

With the benefit of a few years of hindsight, it's possible to hazard a few judgments about what Service Credit Banking in Managed Care did and didn't accomplish—or what it did and didn't prove about the application of the service credit concept to long-term care. At a minimum, the initiative certainly didn't make a strong case that managed care organizations could be relied on as sustainable homes for such programs. After all, only a few of the service credit banking programs launched by The Robert Wood Johnson Foundation grants survived in some form into 2001, and they seemed in various ways to be more the exception than the rule. Leigh Hammer, who ran the Sentara program that didn't make it, argued that it would have been better off housed at a charitable organization with a strong commitment to public service—and therefore a desire to keep up the mission through thick times and thin.

Judith Whang, the Robert Wood Johnson Foundation officer who eventually came to oversee the program, wondered in retrospect whether the Foundation should have waited until the managed care market stabilized before launching the program. "The benefits here were marginal," Whang said in an interview. But she added that that doesn't mean the program was a waste of time or money. "The concept was fascinating enough that it got people to think about launching volunteer programs with different motives," she said. "One of the benefits of a foundation like this is to try ideas and fail—and it's okay."

"You can't point to what we've accomplished as a success," Mark Meiners agreed. "On one level, it bombed," mostly, in his view, because of the way managed care was falling apart across the country. But Meiners was far from willing to call the service credit concept a failure: "I think it's possible that it's not the way to go, although I'm really not ready to say that yet."

So what did the experiment show about the role of service credits? Were they effective in building the sense of community and reciprocity that Edgar Cahn envisioned? The consensus from participants is: yes, and—well—no.

Clearly, in some instances the credits were an attraction that piqued the interest of volunteers and helped induce them to provide their services. Even if they had no intention of ever cashing in the credits, it seems that many volunteers watched their credit balances like hawks. In almost all the programs, volunteers got periodic mailings listing the number of credits they had accrued—and "they would call you if their quarterly summary wasn't correct," Rocky Mountain HMO's Diane Dickey recalled. In her view, the credits functioned as a kind of glue that reinforced the human bonds that underlay the program. "I think you could have a volunteer program without service credits, but it wouldn't have been as successful," she said.

On the other hand, more volunteers than not, it seemed, were like Ted and Rita Rodda, the Colorado time bank volunteers at Rocky Mountain HMO. "The credits never mattered to us," Rita said in an interview—pointing out that, as non-members of the HMO, they could not have cashed in credits to use services. And even Marie Schmalz, who succeeded Diane Dickey at the Rocky Mountain time bank, has her doubts. "As far as I'm concerned, volunteers didn't do it for the credits," she said. "They may have started out doing it for that reason, but you give them a couple of good experiences and they forget about the credit." In other words, credits were at best a kind of hook—a gimmick—to get volunteers in the door. But they certainly didn't keep them there.

Still more evidence supporting this view comes from the one other program that survives out of the original six Service Credit Banking in Managed Care grants. That's CareXchange, the program launched at CareAmerica, an HMO that was bought by BlueShield of California in 1998. As of early 2001, CareXchange had roughly 400 volunteers and 840 service recipients scattered across five Southern California counties. But late in 2000, CareXchange made a crucial decision to dump the service credits and become just a standard-issue volunteer program—one in which volunteers perform services because they want to, and nothing more.

"I really didn't want to give the service credits up," said CareXchange's director, Mindy Morgen, who had written the original proposal to get the grant from The Robert Wood Johnson Foundation and once considered herself highly devoted to the concept. But what underlay the decision to abandon the credits was that administratively "it was a nightmare to manage them," she said. It took considerable amounts of staff time just to manage the banking functions of keeping track of the credits—so much so, in fact, that the program had actually stopped sending out statements of service credit balances to volunteers a few months after it began. Then, in November of 2000, a CareXchange newsletter to participants carried the news that the service credits were being officially dumped as of 2001. "We got no feedback at all" from the program participants, Morgen said. "No one wanted them anymore. No one cared."

So in the final analysis, are service credits or time dollars a concept whose time is coming—or merely a fringe idea, likely to play only the smallest of roles as society confronts the challenge of long-term care? A dispassionate evaluation of The Robert Wood Johnson Foundation experiments might tend to underscore the latter view, since so few of them have survived, and since even they are serving relatively small numbers of elderly people. From this perspective, it seems impossible to imagine a national time dollars program serving anything like the numbers of people likely to need long-term care services in the future. Rather, time dollars could be to long-term care what windmills and solar panels are to the nation's energy supply: a small, unconventional, even noble way of serving the few, but nothing to be relied upon to meet the needs of the masses.

Then there's the alternative view of service credit programs—that their time, if not already here, is coming. In a sense, they fall midway along the spectrum of options available to us as a society for providing long-term care. At one end, we could tax ourselves in order to pay others to provide care for our aging and frail loved ones. At the other extreme, we could freely provide all the care to our loved ones ourselves. In the middle are systems with the sort of dualism Tocqueville would have recognized—partly formal and partly informal caregiving systems, perhaps built around service credits, a kind of oxymoronic payment to reward the altruism of others. In twenty-first century America, where neither of the two aforementioned extremes seems possible, perhaps service credit banking programs could be a practical compromise.

Not surprisingly, the view that service credit banking has a future is shared by Cahn and other enthusiasts helping to run dozens of other time dollar programs around the world. The concept is spreading, Cahn argued, for the same reason other waves of social activism have taken off in the past: because "those involved feel they are somehow at the hub of a movement that can make a real difference in the world." The notion of a community coming together to meet its collective needs "resonates with people of vision because it speaks explicitly to global economics, to social justice issues on multiple levels: pragmatic, day-to-day, spiritual, policy, intellectual."

What's more, said Cahn, if time dollars or service credits didn't already exist, someone would have to invent them—since they are a proxy for the very thing that must be at the crux of long-term care. "I don't think we can crack long-term care in this country until we can figure out a way to create these informal support systems in a way we can depend on," Cahn said. "The operative word is community, which implies stability, but the reality of our present-day existence is flux. The mitigating intermediary is something called memory. If we can figure out a way to create the equivalent of family memory, community memory, institutional memory, we can figure out a way to crack the problem of long-term care." Or to put it another way: if you can build a community by proxy across three boroughs of New York City, as the Elderplan's Member to Member program is doing to this very day, perhaps you really can build it anywhere.

For all of the problems in administering programs built around them, then, service credits, in the best of all worlds, can become a proxy for vanishing memory. Perhaps it is a memory that conjures up for us a time in our Tocquevillian, mythic past when, we believe, people cared for one another more than we do now. It is, in any case, a memory of feelings that we ourselves may have felt as we've helped an ailing neighbor or placed a comforting call to a lonely friend. For it is at those moments that we've understood that we are connected to one another, that the connection matters—and that it will doubtless matter all the more to us as we age.

Notes

1. A. de Tocqueville, *Democracy in America*, R. D. Heffner, ed. (New York: New American Library, 1984), p.198.

2. Ibid, p. 254.

3. National Academy on Aging. *Facts on Long-Term Care, 1997*. Washington, D.C. Available at http://geron.org/NAA/ltc.html.

4. P. S. Arno, C. Levine, and M. M. Memmott, "The Economic Value of Informal Caregiving," *Health Affairs*, 1999, volume 18, number 2, pp. 182–188.

5. R. B. Friedland and L. Summer. *Demography is Not Destiny*. National Academy on an Aging Society, January 1999. Report cites statistics from U.S. Census Bureau, Population Projections of the United States by Age, Race, Sex, Race, and Hispanic Origin: 1995 to 2050, P25–1130, Table F, 1996. Also Census Bureau, 65+ in the United States, P23–190, Table 2-1, 1996.

6. J. Feder, J. Howard, W. Scanlon, "Helping Oneself by Helping Others: Evaluation of a Service Credit Banking Demonstration," *Journal of Aging and Social Policy*, 1992, volume 4, number 3/4, pp. 111–138.

7. Ibid, p. 111.

CHAPTER FIVE

~~~ Consumer Choice in Long-term Care

A. E. Benjamin and Rani E. Snyder

Editors' Introduction

Consumer choice exists for goods and services in most markets, and it can also play a role in long-term care. This concept is attractive to advocates for the rights of people with disabilities, since it enables disabled people themselves to make choices about the services they will receive. At the same time, consumer choice appeals to those who want greater efficiency in government programs, for the individuals whose lives are affected can be expected to choose more wisely than outsiders—such as government officials.

Although this simple concept is gaining in popularity, it is still controversial. Many people believe that older citizens or those with developmental disabilities are not able to make proper choices about their care. There is also concern among traditional home care agencies that disabled people will choose to pay family members, rather than outside agencies, with funds that become available under consumer choice programs.

Beginning in the early 1990s, The Robert Wood Johnson Foundation funded three national programs to test various ways of giving consumers more choice in the services they use and the people who provide them. The first awarded grants to states for programs that enabled people with developmental disabilities to make their own decisions about the care they receive. The second program provided poor elderly people with money to buy home care services, and gave them additional support with such tasks as financial planning and bookkeeping. The third program tested a wide range of approaches to giving people with disabilities greater choice in the kind of care they receive.

In this chapter, A. E. (Ted) Benjamin, the chair of the Department of Social Welfare at the University of California, Los Angeles, and the evaluator of one of the programs, and his colleague Rani Snyder, a research associate and doctoral candidate at UCLA, examine each of the programs and draw preliminary lessons from them.

The Foundation's method of increasing consumer choice in long-term care illustrates three ways it approaches issues. First, it designed a series of programs focused on different aspects of a common theme; the Foundation's size allows it to make very large, mutually reinforcing investments that address a single issue. Second, the three programs focus not on one specific subgroup of the chronically ill; rather, the programs are aimed at groups as diverse as the elderly disabled, the non-elderly disabled, and people with developmental disabilities, many of whom are children. Third, the Foundation timed the initiatives to take advantage of a rising wave of change. In the early 1990s, a number of groups representing disabled people were focusing on the issue of consumer direction. By working with these groups, the Foundation could help shape the direction of the wave and amplify the efforts of others working to increase the choices available to people needing long-term care.

—◦∿◦—

Most people with chronic conditions don't live in nursing homes or hospitals. They live at home or in other community housing. While their medical care is obviously important to them, so is the assistance that allows them to live successfully in their communities. For many people with long-term disabilities, such assistance involves fairly prosaic tasks far removed from medical science and technology—tasks such as help with bathing, dressing, and other routine activities, along with assistance in housekeeping, chores, and transportation. Family members have traditionally taken on these tasks. There is mounting evidence, however, that many people who need assistance live apart from their families, and that many families are not able to manage the demands placed on them by members in need. How can society respond to the needs of frail elderly people and younger people with disabilities in ways that are helpful, sufficient, and cost-effective?[1]

Since the early 1970s, representatives of younger people with disabilities have suggested an innovative approach. They have argued that rather than invest further in agency-based services run by professional nurses and social workers, society should instead channel resources directly to people with disabilities so that they might control the services they need. This argument, which has roots in both the civil rights and consumer movements of the 1960s, suggests that it is a mistake to think that people with disabilities primarily need medical services at home; what they most need is supportive services at home and in their community that do not require medical supervision. So, rather than organize supportive services through medically oriented, professionally run, and expensive home care agencies, what is needed are supportive services programs that rely less on professional staff and procedures and more on the strengths and the preferences of the people in need.[2]

Over the years, a few states such as California, Oregon, and Maine have established home-based supportive services programs based on the principles of consumer control, in which services are authorized and paid for by the state but all or most decisions about whom to hire and which supportive services are provided are made by those who receive the services.[3] While consumer-directed programs for younger people with disabilities are more common than those for older people, some prominent state programs, California's among them, reimburse such services for disabled people of any age.[4] Because professionals and home care agencies play a minor role in such programs, administrative overhead is relatively low, and a higher percentage of resources are devoted to services that go directly to those in need.[5] These programs have nonetheless been the targets of persistent criticism: How can we spend public funds without professional scrutiny and accountability? How can recipient safety be assured without professional oversight? How can we know that service needs are being met without professional monitoring? How can we be sure that frail older people are as able as younger disabled people to assume the demands of self-direction?

Despite such concerns, having consumers direct their own home care is an idea that no longer resides on the fringes; it has become a mainstream part of long-term care policy debates. Even with its anti-professional rhetoric, the theme of consumer direction has begun to appear regularly on the agendas of professional meetings and in articles published in professional journals.

⁓ One Theme, Three Programs

Chronic care has been a priority of The Robert Wood Johnson Foundation since 1991. Before then, Foundation funding initiatives had targeted issues related to a few specific chronic diseases like AIDS and Alzheimer's. Early in the 1990s, Foundation staff members recommended a broader approach to the challenges that seemed common to these and other chronic conditions, namely to redirect the thinking about chronic services to go beyond treatment of acute illness provided by physicians and toward the development of community care that would expand the choices available to people with chronic impairments. While many policymakers tended to equate issues of chronic, or long-term, care with elderly people, Foundation staff members had already been made aware of the diversity of people who needed long-term care services.

In 1990, the Foundation announced a series of grants to independent living centers under a program called Improving Service Systems for People with Disabilities. Independent living centers are local nonprofit organizations, typically run by younger adults with physical disabilities, that advocate for and provide services to disabled people. This small initiative encouraged the centers to explore new ideas for improving services and for strengthening the networks that provided them. More important, perhaps, the program served as an introduction for the Foundation to the Independent Living Movement, whose leaders, themselves people with disabilities, emphasized two themes: first, expanding public support for services to help younger adults with physical disabilities live independently and productively in their communities; and, second, developing and disseminating models that emphasized consumer choice and control over core services that are considered essential to independent living—most notably, personal assistance.

In 1995, the Foundation joined with the federal Administration on Aging and the Assistant Secretary for Planning and Evaluation of the U.S. Department of Health and Human Services to establish the National Institute on Consumer-Directed Long-Term Services to bring together representatives of older people (the National Council on the Aging) and younger people (the World Institute on Disability). The idea was that these representatives could foster increased opportunities for consumer choice and direction in services for adults with disabilities. The collaboration produced a document that addressed the basics of this approach and provided a definition of the key elements of consumer direction:

> Consumer direction is a philosophy and orientation to the delivery of home and community-based services whereby informed consumers make choices about the services they receive. They can assess their own needs, determine how and by whom these needs should be met, and monitor the quality of services received. Consumer direction may exist in differing degrees and may span many types of services. It ranges from the individual independently making all decisions and managing services directly, to an individual using a representative to manage needed services. The unifying force in the range of . . . models is that individuals have the primary authority to make choices that work best for them, regardless of the nature or extent of their disability or the source of the payment for services.[6]

In 1995, the Foundation also launched three initiatives designed to strengthen the role of disabled consumers in shaping decisions about their own lives. Each of the initiatives supported consumer-directed service models for different disabled populations. Because of the variety of constituencies—elderly people, young adults with disabilities, developmentally disabled people, children with special health care needs, the chronically mentally ill, and others—and the range of separate funding systems, each with distinctive constraints, designing a single initiative was simply not considered realistic. The three initiatives were Self-Determination for Persons with Developmental Disabilities, Cash and Counseling, and Independent Choices: Enhancing Consumer Direction for People with Disabilities.

~~~ The Self-Determination for Persons with Developmental Disabilities Program

Lynn is a young woman who was paralyzed from the neck down in a childhood accident. Although her disabilities were physical, she had been declared incompetent and confined to a nursing home for years. She was contacted by people from Wayne County's Health and Community Services in Michigan and was asked for the first time since her accident what she wanted to see happen with her life. After identifying people she wanted in her support circle, she was given a budget (drawing from Medicaid funds that would have gone to the nursing home) and assisted in planning her life outside the institution. She arranged to hire a personal assistant and found a home to rent. The home was modified to accommodate her disabilities. She later persuaded a male friend she had met in the nursing home to share the house with her; he too has a fund drawn from Medicaid that he manages for himself. Lynn now has a new life and the freedom to plan and dream for the future and has been able to arrange the supports she needs to manage her own life.[7]

Arthur is a 54-year-old man with a developmental disability who had lived with his (now aging) parents all his life. After looking at group homes and finding them unappealing, Arthur became part of a new program at the Hudson Valley Developmental Disability Service Organization in New York State. Arthur enlisted family members to work with him and his service coordinator in finding an apartment that met his needs and that allowed him easy access to his job at the local YM/YWCA. He was able to use his service fund to hire someone to help him shop and cook and to hire others to assist him in learning to budget and to use a computer. Arthur hopes to develop computer skills that will get him a better job; for now, he communicates with his support circle via e-mail. Recently, after an arduous process, he was able to purchase the co-op unit in which he had been living. Arthur is now a proud home owner.[8]

Lynn and Arthur are two participants in a Robert Wood Johnson Foundation–funded program called Self-Determination for Persons with Developmental Disabilities. The roots of this program can be traced back to the deinstitutionalization movement of the 1960s and 1970s, when community living had become a major theme among advocates for people with developmental disabilities. In state and federal policy debates, families had been arguing that they, rather than mental health services professionals, should be making basic decisions about how family members with developmental disabilities should live. In reality, the dominant option for many families had become the "intermediate care facility—mental retardation." These facilities generally had 15 or more beds and provided residential and supportive services. State Medicaid programs pay dearly for this care, approaching $100,000 a year per resident. States had also developed programs, funded under Medicaid waivers, tailored to meet individual needs of people with developmental disabilities in their homes or communities. Trends toward community living and stronger consumer roles for those with developmental disabilities were also fueled by passage of the federal Community Supported Living Arrangements Act in 1990, which funded supported living projects in up to eight states for those who would otherwise need to be placed in intermediate care facilities.[9]

In 1993, The Robert Wood Johnson Foundation funded a small pilot project in community living in New Hampshire called the Monadnock Self-Determination for People with Developmental Disabilities Project. In the project, a case manager worked with individuals—mainly those who had been institutionalized in state facilities—and their friends and families to develop a plan for procuring needed services in the community. Not long after, the founders of Monadnock brought to the Foundation a proposal to expand the approach and develop a larger community service system designed by people with developmental disabilities and their circle of friends.

The Robert Wood Johnson Foundation authorized a $5 million, three-year program called Self-Determination for Persons with Developmental Disabilities in October, 1995 and issued a Call for Proposals in 1996. The program guidelines encouraged states to create new and enhanced opportunities for developmentally disabled people to choose what support and services they would receive, how they would live in their communities, and where they would find jobs or other meaningful roles. Self-determination is based on the principles of freedom, authority, support, and responsibility:[10]

- *Freedom*: the ability of disabled people to choose those making up their support system, to decide where and with whom they want to live, and to determine with whom they choose to spend their time. They may select family members or friends to help them.

- *Authority*: the ability, with help as needed, to make all decisions about support and to control funds in order to buy needed services; it includes the ability to modify priorities over time.

- *Support*: needed by many developmentally disabled people to take responsibility for decisionmaking and to live fully in the community, yet it must truly be support—not supervision. People with disabilities may wish to rely on family, friends, or one or more contracts for help with discrete tasks.

- *Responsibility*: the notion that public dollars must be used wisely.

Through the Self-Determination program, grants were made to 19 states. Additional sites in ten other states were chosen for smaller technical assistance grants. Thus, more than half the 50 states have been engaged in assessing the status of their current systems of care for developmentally disabled people and exploring new options aimed at helping them shape their own lives. At the heart of the Self-Determination program is the direct involvement of people with developmental disabilities in planning and overseeing implementation of their service systems: from making policy and serving as members of advisory boards to preparing their own plans and budgets. Each of the 29 projects shares three features. Plans are developed by users and their support groups, and budgets controlled by the users. They provide for monitoring by state project teams to insure that people with disabilities identify and obtain the individually tailored supports they want. And each project provides for administrative support—a state, for example, might contract with fiscal agents to assist local projects and recipients in developing and managing individual budgets—so that state systems work effectively.

A project in Massachusetts illustrates how the Self-Determination program works. In the Boston area, the project created family governing boards to represent major ethnic groups in the community, including Haitian, Asian, Latin American, and Ethiopian populations. The governing boards generally consist of six to eight families, overall representing more than 500 families. They meet on a quarterly basis. Most of the boards are linked with community agencies (rather than traditional mental retardation agencies), and the community agency hires a staff on behalf of the families. The boards are charged with working together to determine how the mix of state and federal funds are spent. The money is pooled rather than individually allocated.

One important element of this arrangement is that the contracts are between the family governing board, rather than a government agency, and the providers of services. Knowing that choices and payments are controlled by the family governing board, the providers of services must be responsive to the boards and the consumers. This strategy invites more family and community involvement than has historically taken place. As news of this initiative spreads through the community, more families have come forward to participate in the process.

⁓ The Rationale Behind the Cash and Counseling and Independent Choices Programs

While a network of independent living centers, financed by Medicaid or state funds, and other programs giving choices to physically disabled young people have existed since the 1970s, those who represent older Americans have been slower to warm to the idea of self-direction, believing that older people are less interested in and less capable of directing their own services. As a result, experience with older consumers and self-direction has been comparatively limited.[11] In the last decade, however, influential individuals such as James Firman, who is executive director of the National Council on the Aging (and who, in the past, was a program officer at The Robert Wood Johnson Foundation), have been calling for expanded consumer choice in service programs for elderly people. Across age groups, advocates have called for providing recipients with cash rather than services; that is, turning over the direct control of service funds to eligible people with disabilities to use as they wish, typically within some constraints. Others have suggested that most people, including the very old, would welcome more control over their home and community services but may be hesitant about directly handling and accounting for public funds.

In this context, in 1995 the Foundation authorized two programs to support a range of approaches to expanding consumer direction: Cash and Counseling, a four-year program approved at a $2.1 million level, and Independent Choices, a four-year program approved at a $3.4 million level.[12] In both programs, the Foundation also wanted to understand what happens when consumer direction is extended to elderly people.

The first approach was the cash model, offering consumers a cash allowance in lieu of services provided by social agencies. It was expected to provide the maximum of flexibility in services by leaving most decisions to the consumer and to reduce overall costs by minimizing professional services, such as those provided by home care agencies. There was some concern, however, that a cash program alone was not enough; people might need assistance in getting started as their own case managers. Thus was born the idea of Cash and Counseling—of giving control of resources to the recipients and providing support they needed to deal with expanded choices. In the second approach, the Foundation authorized a broader initiative that would support various innovative approaches, apart from cash, for fostering choice and control in long-term care. This was called Independent Choices.

⸺ The Cash and Counseling Program

The Cash and Counseling program was based on careful background analysis. The Foundation had commissioned a study of programs in other countries that permitted long-term care recipients to choose between cash benefits and information services, vouchers, and traditional case-managed, agency-based services. This study had found that cash and counseling programs were popular in other countries and seemed to save money when compared with traditional programs. What was now being proposed was a large-scale demonstration and a rigorous evaluation in this country. The idea had also attracted the attention of federal officials, and the Office of the Assistant Secretary for Planning and Evaluation within the U.S. Department of Health and Human Services offered to contribute a significant share of the evaluation costs. In early 1996, a national program office at the University of Maryland Center on Aging began soliciting proposals from states interested in setting up demonstration programs.

Four states—Arkansas, Florida, New Jersey, and New York—were chosen from among seventeen that applied for funds. In late 1998, the programs began in three of those states; for a variety of reasons, New York was dropped from the demonstration. While many details vary, the basic design is the same in all three states. Consumers are Medicaid-eligible adults who qualify for personal assistance services because of significant functional limitations with activities of daily living, such as bathing, dressing, toileting, or eating. They are offered a choice between receiving home care services or cash allowances to buy these services themselves. The value of each cash allowance is set at approximately the cost of the traditional care plan. (Because this is designed as an experiment, those who choose the cash allowance are randomly assigned to cash or to traditional services.) Those who get the cash allowance can also receive counseling services and assistance with fiscal tasks and bookkeeping. Counselors are available to help the participants develop a cash plan, locate, train and manage workers, gain access to community resources, and develop a backup plan.[13] The participants in the program are required to spend their allowance on their personal assistance needs. They can return to the traditional program at any time.

Although the evaluation of the Cash and Counseling program will not be completed until 2003, early analysis from the three states

---

♪♪♪

Ms. F. lives alone at age 92. Recently recovered from broken bones and surgery to implant a heart pacemaker, she is determined to remain independent and does as much for herself as possible. She uses her Cash and Counseling allowance to pay her daughter to help her and be available when needed, especially when she gets ready for church and visits to the senior center. She use some of the allowance to purchase personal care supplies and over-the-counter medications.

reveals some interesting lessons. If the cash option is carefully presented, many frail elderly people and others eligible for personal assistance services traditionally provided by agencies are willing to try it.[14] The vast majority of enrollees choose to hire a family member or a friend as a paid provider. Most enrollees choose to have a state-contracted "fiscal intermediary" handle employer and bookkeeping tasks, thus easing state concerns about accountability and liability. Early experience also suggests that the small number of enrollees who want to perform these tasks themselves can be trained to do them adequately. In Arkansas, recipients may use some of their monthly cash allowance for items other than personal assistance services. In that state, most funds were used to pay workers for direct home-based services, but about one in six dollars went to buy or repair equipment related to their care and safety or to do modest home modifications.[15]

Some of the program challenges involve people other than those who receive services. For example, it has proven difficult to teach case managers to market the cash option to their clients and to become non-directive counselors and consultants. Also, home care workers must be educated about the new options, since they may view consumer direction as a threat to their employment. Overall, there is more to be learned about how people regard the cash option, how well workers and case managers adapt to their new roles, and the types and amounts of counseling assistance that are most needed.

꽃

Ms. M is a very large person in her 80's who needs assistance with most activities. She has had a difficult time arranging for agency home care, because workers prefer clients with fewer needs. Ms. M. has used her Cash and Counseling allowance to hire a granddaughter to assist with personal care tasks like bathing and dressing and also to pay a grandson to stay with her in the evenings when her daughter (with whom she lives) is away. She is saving any unspent funds to make payments on the badly needed dentures she bought after entering the program.

⌁ The Independent Choices Program

Independent Choices was designed to complement the Cash and Counseling program by supporting smaller-scale demonstration projects and research. Both programs seek to advance consumer choice in long-term care services. Unlike the Cash and Counseling approach, which tested a single strategy in different locations across the country, the Independent Choices program used a portfolio approach, with individual projects chosen to address diverse populations and different concepts. The broader approach has allowed the Foundation to fund a continuum of consumer-directed models in a variety of settings, but has precluded a standardized evaluation of the program, since each project was highly individual. Although this approach makes it harder to assess program impact, it also opens the door to a range of projects designed to move the concept of consumer direction more into the mainstream.

The National Council on the Aging has served as the National Program Office for the Independent Choices initiative. It was charged with helping to identify and develop projects that would represent the full spectrum of challenges facing consumer-directed home and community-based services for people of all ages with chronic disabilities. The Foundation issued a Call for Proposals in 1996 to develop and test approaches other than the cash option to empower the consumers of long-term care. To the surprise of almost everyone, nearly 500 applications for Independent Choices funding were received. In the summer of 1997, the National Council on the Aging selected thirteen sites for funding.

Of these sites, four were research projects and nine were demonstrations. The four research projects were chosen to increase understanding about people's preferences for consumer direction and how these preferences might differ across consumer groups. The nine demonstration projects have focused on new approaches to delivering consumer-directed care for different population groups.

At the Family Caregiver Alliance in San Francisco, for example, a study was fielded to understand more about how people with mild to moderate cognitive impairment might adapt to consumer-directed services. How well do people with cognitive limitations express their own preferences, and how consistently do they present them over time? How well do the views of family members reflect the preferences of their cognitively impaired relatives?

Project staff members conducted three lengthy interviews with each of 50 pairs of clients and primary caregivers. The results of these interviews indicated that people with mild to moderate cognitive impairment could reliably answer questions about demographics, general life style preferences, health care preferences, and making decisions. They answered factual questions accurately and consistently and expressed specific wishes and values. Since most clients had family members helping them in their lives, it was surprising to find numerous differences between what family members thought their relatives with cognitive impairment valued in the way of services and what those people themselves valued. In effect, those with mild to moderate cognitive impairments could express their preferences clearly and consistently, and family members were imperfect spokespersons for them. The findings open up more possibilities for consumer direction to be tailored to those with cognitive problems but, at the same time, are distressing because the system relies so heavily on family members to speak for those who are judged unable to speak for themselves.[16]

Another research project, at the Schneider Institute for Health Policy at Brandeis University, was designed to examine the preferences of older disabled Bostonians about self-direction in long-term care services, and whether those preferences varied by race or ethnicity. Staff members for this project conducted face-to-face interviews with 731 low-income elderly persons with chronic illness or disability who were already receiving home care services through various state and local programs, none of which offered the option of services directed by the consumer. Four separate populations of elderly people were interviewed: African-American, Chinese-American, Latino, and Western European. While the results are still being analyzed, they indicate that there are significant differences based on race or ethnicity in elder preferences regarding consumer direction. For example, when given different options, elderly Chinese and African-Americans are more likely to select the cash and counseling option than are elders in the other two groups. Researchers are exploring the reasons for these differences, but this study has already laid the groundwork for understanding how cultural differences can influence the way different groups respond to different service arrangements.

Among the demonstration projects supported by Independent Choices, three are designed to expand the options available to those who use Medicaid's long-term home care services, especially elderly people. The most ambitious are programs in Ohio and Oregon that are attempting to expand the options available to the people receiving care. In Ohio, a project team at Miami University is working with a regional Area Agency on Aging and with the state Department on Aging to expand the options available to elders in central Ohio whose services are provided under an existing "waiver program" (these programs must receive approval from the federal government to waive existing federal Medicaid regulations in order to provide services in innovative ways). The plan is to teach current and prospective recipients what the specific options are and how to make them work, and then let those recipients choose how they want their services designed: traditional case-managed services; modified case management, in which the consumer has more authority; or a consumer-directed option involving hiring and managing their own workers. However, the initiative has encountered problems in convincing the federal government to modify an existing waiver in order to add more consumer-directed options to the service menu.

Oregon has long offered innovative home-based and community-based services with some features chosen by recipients, and under Independent Choices the state is attempting to expand the choices available under its "client-employed provider program." Along with offering recipients a wider selection of providers and the opportunity to use their cash benefits for tasks not previously covered, the most significant new step is giving them, and not the state, responsibility for paying providers and payroll taxes. Rather than assuming that most recipients need accounting services, Oregon has argued that many of them can learn to handle the bookkeeping tasks associated with being an employer. Like Ohio and Minnesota (and a number of other Independent Choices sites), Oregon has emphasized the development of training to prepare consumers for self-direction. Oregon and the other sites are also targeting case managers, providers, and family members for training, since everyone's role is altered when the consumer is the primary decision maker about services.

Other demonstration sites, such as Forest Park, Illinois, and Oakland, California, are tackling related challenges. The Progress Center for Independent Living in Forest Park, Illinois, is forging alliances with home care agencies to help educate them about consumer direction and enable them to become collaborators in expanding consumer roles. Under current Medicaid waiver programs in Illinois, disabled people over age 60 can receive home-based services only through an agency, while those under age 60 must hire their own workers with help from programs like the Progress Center for Independent Living. Through this Independent Choices project, the staff members are attempting not only to win support from skeptical home health agencies but also to build bridges between younger and older disabled people by demonstrating how home health care agencies can be converted to the idea of consumer direction. In part because the home care industry is in such turmoil as a result of expansions in managed care and recent cuts in reimbursement, finding agency collaborators and nurturing working relationships with them is proving much more difficult than expected.

A public agency in Oakland, California, has developed emergency backup services for people with disabilities who suddenly find themselves without assistance. Medicaid in California provides personal assistance services to nearly 200,000 people, and most of them hire, train, and supervise their own home care workers with little or no outside assistance. One critical problem involves backup; that is, what happens when a worker someone depends on for assistance in basic activities like dressing, toileting, and eating is sick or otherwise unable to work? The Oakland program has created an emergency assistance hotline to fill this gap.[17]

ॐ

Mrs. Y is a 72-year-old woman who lives alone and has limited vision because of her diabetes. One morning, Mrs. Y's regularly scheduled worker did not arrive to assist her. Mrs. Y was alarmed because she requires meals and snacks at specific times, and she had not been bathed in several days. Mrs. Y was able to call the new program, called Rapid Response, and a substitute worker arrived within one hour. She discussed with Mrs. Y the tasks to be done and then proceeded to prepare her meals, assist with bathing, and pick up needed groceries.

—— Lessons Learned

Since many of the sites are still putting these initiatives in place and evaluating them, the lessons of the three programs are not yet fully understood. Even as more formal evaluations of these programs are being completed, some general conclusions can be drawn about their initial impact.

> *First, these programs have stimulated interest in the idea of consumer choice in long-term care.*

Although some formidable barriers still confront broad dissemination, the programs are helping to position the idea of consumer choice more firmly in the mainstream, and are altering the debate. Ideologically charged questions are still being asked about whether expanded consumer choice is desirable or feasible, but attention is now being paid to more pragmatic questions about which forms of self-direction work best and under which circumstances. In other words, the long-term care field seems to have moved from issues of "why?" to issues of "how?"

> *Second, while barriers do remain in extending consumer-directed services to elderly people, there is also a growing consensus that at least a substantial minority of those over age 65 want to give consumer-direction a chance.*

While numerous skeptics exist, many experts now acknowledge that there are few, if any, age-defined barriers to making consumer choice work for elderly people. While younger adults continue to be the most fervent advocates for expanded consumer choice, growing numbers of organizations that represent the aging have now joined the chorus. The National Council on the Aging, which had long backed consumer direction, became a more active and visible proponent since the Independent Choices program's inception.

> *Third, even if the idea of introducing consumer direction to people with cognitive disabilities may seem unrealistic, people with solid research and program credentials now report that it is feasible.*

The developmentally disabled community has devised self-determination options that seem to work for a range of people with developmental disabilities. Younger people accustomed to making their own choices are likely to demand the same options as they themselves become elderly. In a sense, the last frontier in the extension of consumer choice is older people with cognitive limitations. Both research and experience suggest that these people, too, can exercise choice if given appropriate support.

Fourth, the programs have clarified the challenges in translating ideas about consumer choice into tangible program options.

In considering which people to enroll, most sites in the three programs have rejected screening clients and including only the most promising. Instead, sites have decided to enroll anyone who meets the program's disability requirements and then to provide them with whatever resources they need to support expanded choice. In sites with a cash option, this has often meant providing fiscal and accounting services. Other support includes training about consumer direction, assistance in finding a worker, and help with arranging a backup plan. More basically, program sites are demonstrating that a universal approach—a non-screening approach—seems feasible.

Related to this is the issue of representation. People with debilitating physical conditions—and especially those with cognitive disabilities—are typically believed to need routine assistance or supervision not only in basic life activities but also in making decisions. The family frequently assumes the role of representative for the person with disability when dealing with service systems and making service choices. All three programs recognize the importance of families and incorporate them into the process, while also recognizing that the preferences and interests of the family are not always identical with those of the person with disabilities. Even before the findings from the Family Caregiver Alliance study became available, most sites were committed to giving people with disabilities maximum independence while using family resources to further that end. (The sites for the most part have resisted surrogacy models, in which a family member or another designated representative speaks for the person with disability. This model seems most appealing where elderly people with Alzheimer's are involved.) The challenge has been to encourage the supportive character of family collaboration while also acknowledging the primacy of consumer interests.

Fifth, if any one set of activities characterizes these three programs, it is training.

While training in home care has traditionally been aimed at preparing workers to address the needs of clients, these programs have focused on training people to understand and implement consumer-directed services and on providing them with needed support. People unfamiliar with self-direction are one target: much work has been done to design and disseminate training materials for those with diverse needs—those who are illiterate, for example. Other target audiences include family members, service providers, case managers, independent brokers, and others providing services needed by people with disabilities.

Sixth, the programs have furthered a reconsideration of case management.

The term "case management" is not popular among those who support consumer direction. A frequent response to the term is "I am not a case, and I do not want to be managed." Yet case management is widely practiced and valued in professional circles and in public programs. Traditionally, case managers are trained to make decisions for clients after consulting with them and their families. Various sites have been working to retrain case managers to think differently about consumer roles and to incorporate consumer-directed options as they assess and enroll new clients. This has been an uphill battle. Some sites have screened case managers to identify those who are most open to consumer direction and then assigned only these people to key program roles. Others are testing the feasibility of a broader approach that attempts to reorient all case managers working with elderly and younger people with disabilities. It remains uncertain whether professionals whose early training and orientation is founded on conceptions of client dependency, dysfunction, and need can be persuaded to revise their assumptions and give more choice to the people who receive the services.

—— Looking Ahead

Ideas about consumer choice are now part of the mainstream discussion on the future of long-term care services for people who are aged or disabled. While not long ago many states viewed elderly people as indifferent to these options, they are now analyzing and implementing options that put authority into the hands of those who are receiving services. Rather than simply asking whether it is possible, there is now more focus on how to make consumer direction work by making it possible for people to find their own workers, arrange backup, and deal with decisionmaking issues. Even with this progress, however, major challenges remain to be met.

Approaches that shift decisions about resources are certain to stimulate resistance. Disabled consumers, who depend heavily on current services to improve their lives, are often wary of changes that might alter familiar arrangements. They worry not only about change itself but also about possible cuts in benefits and about assuming added responsibilities. Established home care agencies worry about lost business and revenues. The network for aging services is concerned about losing control over resources, and about losing the political influence that goes with them. Budget watchers concerned with public accountability worry about fraud and abuse. Consumer direction seems like a reasonable option to those troubled by the shortage of workers willing to do home care, since it may help expand the pool by letting people hire friends and family. To others, choice seems more untenable than the current situation since consumers themselves must find scarce workers or risk going without services.

Despite the barriers, consumer direction now has the attention of a much broader range of federal and state agencies, policy and program officials, and academic researchers than was the case previously. There is much more experimenting, knowledge is increasing, and consumer direction is moving from being a radical approach for younger disabled people to being a mainstream option for all people with disabilities.

Notes

1. A. E. Benjamin, "An Historical Perspective on Home Care Policy," *The Milbank Quarterly*, 1993, volume 71, pp. 129–166.
2. C. W. Mahoney, C. L. Estes, and J. E. Heumann, *Toward A Unified Agenda: Proceedings of a National Conference on Disability and Aging* (San Francisco, California: Institute for Health and Aging, 1986); and G. DeJong, A.I. Batavia, and L. B. McKnew, "The Independent Living Model of Personal Assistance in National Long-Term Care Policy," *Generations*, 1992, volume 16, pp. 89–95.

3. P. Doty, J. Kasper, and S. Litvak, "Consumer-Directed Models of Personal Care: Lessons from Medicaid," *The Milbank Quarterly*, 1996, volume 74, pp. 377–409.

4. A. E. Benjamin and R. E. Matthias, "Comparing Consumer- and Agency-Directed Models: California's In-Home Supportive Services Program," *Generations*, 2000, volume 24, pp. 85–87; A. E. Benjamin, R. E. Matthias and T. M. Franke, "Comparing Consumer- Directed and Agency Models for Providing Supportive Services at Home," *Health Services Research*, 2000, volume 35, pp. 351–366.

5. A. I. Batavia, G. DeJong, and L. B. McKnew, "Toward a National Personal Assistance Program: The Independent Living Model of Long-Term Care for Persons with Disabilities," *Journal of Health Politics, Policy and Law*, 1991, volume 16, pp. 523–545.

6. National Institute on Consumer-Directed Long-Term Services, *Principles of Consumer-Directed Home and Community-Based Services* (Washington, DC: National Council on the Aging, Inc. and World Institute on Disability, July 1996).

7. National Program Office on Self-Determination, *Common Sense*, July 1999, issue 4.

8. National Program Office on Self-Determination, *Common Sense*, July 2000, issue 7.

9. K. C. Lakin, "Persons with Developmental Disabilities: Mental Retardation as an Exemplar," in R. J. Newcomer and A. E. Benjamin, editors, *Indicators of Chronic Health Conditions: Monitoring Community-Level Delivery Systems* (Baltimore, Maryland: The Johns Hopkins University Press, 1997).

10. T. Nerney and D. Shumway, *Beyond Managed Care: Self-Determination for People with Disabilities* (Concord, New Hampshire: Institute on Disability, September 1996).

11. N. N. Eustis and L. R. Fischer, "Common Needs, Different Solutions? Younger and Older Homecare Clients," *Generations*, 1992, volume 16, pp. 17–23; L. Simon-Rusinowitz and B. F. Hofland, "Adopting a Disability Approach to Home Care Services for Older Adults," *The Gerontologist*, 1993, volume 33, pp. 159–167.

12. The authorization for Cash and Counseling was increased by $2.83 million in 1996, for a total authorization of $4.93 million. This includes funds for the demonstrations and evaluation.

13. K. J. Mahoney, K. Simone, L. Simon-Rusinowitz, "Early Lessons from the Cash and Counseling Demonstration and Evaluation," *Generations*, 2000, volume 24, pp. 41–46.

14. L. Simon-Rusinowitz, K. J. Mahoney, S. M. Desmond, et al., "Determining Consumer Preferences for a Cash Option: Arkansas Survey Results," *Health Care Financing Review*, 1997, volume 19, pp. 73–96.

15. K. J. Mahoney, K. Simone, L. Simon-Rusinowitz, "Early Lessons from the Cash and Counseling Demonstration and Evaluation," *Generations*, 2000, volume 24, pp. 41–46; and Mathematica Policy Research, Inc., "Issue Brief: Cash and Counseling: Early Experiences in Arkansas," December 2000, number 1.

16. L. F. Feinberg, C. J. Whitlatch, and S. Tucke, *Making Hard Choices; Hearing Both Voices*, final report to The Robert Wood Johnson Foundation (San Francisco, California: Family Caregiver Alliance, May 2000).

17. D. Wong, "Rapid Response: Development of a Homecare Worker Replacement Service," *Generations*, 2000, volume 24, pp. 88–90.

CHAPTER SIX

~~ The Health Policy Fellowships Program

Richard S. Frank

Editors' Introduction

The Health Policy Fellowships Program is one of the Foundation's oldest programs, spanning nearly three decades. It provides one-year fellowships for physicians and other health care professionals to work on health policy issues in Washington, D.C., generally on Capitol Hill.

Only two other major Foundation initiatives can match the longevity of the Health Policy Fellowships Program: The Clinical Scholars Program, the Foundation's postdoctoral training program for young physicians interested in careers in health services research, and the National Health Policy Forum, a Capitol Hill seminar series, co-funded with a number of foundations, which enables Congressional staff members to discuss health policy topics with a range of experts.

The Health Policy Fellowships Program illustrates a primary Foundation strategy of investing in people who are then expected to play leadership roles improving health care, health policy, and public health. Over its history, the program has had other goals, such as increasing the ability of academic medical centers—the professional homes of many of the fellows—to negotiate the world of public policy and to tap the expertise of bright young medical professionals to improve public policy itself.

In this chapter, Richard Frank, the former editor of the *National Journal*, offers a historical overview of the Health Policy Fellowships Program from its inception through its most recent reauthorization, in the spring of 2001. In the process, he describes how the program works, how it has changed over the years, and how some of the Fellows view their experience. Building on external evaluations of the program and interviews with key participants, Frank examines how well the initiative has achieved four different types of objectives. He also discusses some of the critical issues raised by the Health Policy Fellowships Program (and other fellowship programs), such as how to evaluate success and whether the achievements outweigh the high costs.

W hen David P. Stevens arrived in Washington in the fall of 1995, he was looking forward to the beginning of a year as a Health Policy Fellow. He had just taken a year's sabbatical from his post as vice-dean of the Case Western Reserve University School of Medicine, where a year before he had started a program that required medical students to study health policy along with the standard medical courses. As part of the program, the students had to take a two-month Washington internship with a member of Congress or with an advocacy organization. "I believe that physicians of the future must lead change in a formal way, and there is no way you can do that unless you understand the process," Stevens later explained to *The Chronicle of Higher Education.*[1] And now he was about to follow his own prescription.

For the better part of a year, Stevens worked in the office of then-Senator Nancy Landon Kassebaum, the Kansas Republican who headed the Labor and Human Resources Committee, on a variety of legislation, including a bill to reform the system of medical insurance. And as the fellowship entered its final months in the spring of 1996, Stevens was looking forward to returning to the Cleveland campus in September. He intended, he told *The Chronicle* reporter, to put even more emphasis on teaching health policy to his medical school students.

But Stevens never returned to Case Western Reserve. The dean under whom he had served had left the university while Stevens was in Washington, and though Stevens was invited to return, "it was a different set of circumstances," he said in a recent interview, involving the kind of "institutional politics" that occurs whenever there are changes in campus leadership. Instead, he moved to the federal Department of Veterans Affairs for three years as chief of academic affiliations, and he is currently vice-president for medical school standards and assessments at the Association of American Medical Colleges.

Stevens's experience in Washington—"It was enormously valuable," he said—together with his frustrated plans for reforming the academic medical system, echo in some important ways the gratification and the difficulties that the Health Policy Fellowships Program has experienced almost from the day it began in the spring of 1973.

The program, initiated only a year after its sponsor, The Robert Wood Johnson Foundation, became a major national philanthropic foundation, has endured significant revisions in some of its initial goals, along with the recognition that some of those objectives were impossible to achieve and needed to be abandoned. That the Health Policy Fellowships Program is still flourishing, more than a quarter of a century after its conception, is, if nothing else, testimony to the Foundation's pragmatism and flexibility. But at the same time it is a lesson in how easily the reach of an ambitious, policy-oriented foundation can exceed its grasp.

Since the Health Policy Fellowships Program began, it has selected six mid-career physicians and other health care professionals each year—most of them from academic faculties—and sent them to Washington for three months of intensive orientation in how the federal government operates, followed by nine months of full-time service as aides to members of Congress or to congressional committees involved in formulating national health policy or, less frequently, to executive branch officers in the same policy area. Through the end of 2000, 170 Fellows have participated, at a cost to the Foundation of $16.3 million.

The intention, at least at the outset, was "to provide outstanding mid-career health professionals working in academic settings with a better understanding of the major issues in health policy and a knowledge of how federal health policies are established in the United States."[2] The expectation was that these men and women, wise in the ways of Washington, might take senior health policy positions in the federal government while also bringing their newly acquired knowledge and political savvy to bear on their institutions, the academic medical centers that dominate health care in the United States. Underlying these goals was the feeling on the part of the Foundation's leaders that the academic centers needed to change and that the Health Policy Fellows would return to their institutions and take on the role of change agents.

—— Dr. Smith Goes to Washington

The first six Health Policy Fellows were picked in February of 1974 and arrived in Washington that September. Every year since then, another half a dozen men and women have come to the capital as Health Policy Fellows.

Under the auspices of the Institute of Medicine, a branch of the National Academy of Sciences, the Fellows are exposed, during their initial three-month training program, to more than 130 organized briefing sessions as well as meetings with White House aides, heads of relevant federal agencies, leaders of think tanks and interest groups and staff members from the major health committees and subcommittees of the House and Senate. They also participate in seminars on health economics, the congressional budget process, and the federal decision-making process and politics. These sessions are augmented by occasional trips outside of Washington and end with an intensive five-week series of orientation programs that the American Political Science Association conducts for its Congressional Fellowship Program and also makes available to the Health Policy Fellows. "The orientation experience was a rapid yet complete induction into the Washington world of health policy," said Thomas B. Valuck, a 1998–99 Fellow, who is now the vice-president of external affairs at the University of Kansas Medical Center, in his end-of-fellowship evaluation of the program.

A glance at the orientation schedules for recent classes of Fellows bears out Valuck's description. On a typical day, the Fellows might begin at 9:00 a.m. a few blocks from the program's Georgetown headquarters with a 90-minute briefing on the Urban Institute's health-related activities. Next they might travel to the heart of Washington's lobbying community for an hour-long discussion of major issues facing the pharmaceutical industry. Then back to Georgetown for lunch with an alumnus of the program. Finally, the Fellows might cross the Potomac to Alexandria, Virginia, for a two-hour briefing on the agenda of the Institute for Alternative Futures. On another day, the Fellows might spend almost eight hours in a seminar on health policy conducted by a former director of the federal agency that runs Medicare and Medicaid.

All this is preparation, of course, for the heart of the fellowship: the assignment to a congressional or executive branch office. Alumni of the program have described the process of choosing an assignment as turbulent and stressful, according to a team of outside experts who evaluated the program almost a decade ago. To those evaluators, the placement process resembled "a crude marketplace," in which "Fellows seem to find their way to offices that need and want them. . . ." As the program's World Wide Web site describes the process, the Fellows, during the latter stage of the orientation, meet as a group and individually with congressional or executive branch officials active in health issues and, in consultation with the program's director, Marion Ein Lewin of the Institute of Medicine, "negotiate" their assignments. Senate assignments, it turns out, are far more popular than House placements. For the past seven years, all of the Fellows went to work in Senate offices.

The first group—the class of 1974–75—included a psychiatry professor at an East Coast medical school, a professor of family and community medicine and assistant vice-chancellor for academic affairs at a state university on the West Coast, the chairman of the pediatrics department at an East Coast medical school, an associate professor of the history of medicine and public health at another East Coast academic medical center, a member of the faculty at a Southern medical school, and a medical researcher at still another East Coast medical school. All but the assistant vice-chancellor were physicians, though later classes included dentists, registered nurses, and others in the academic community.

In fact, the six Fellows selected each year were chosen exclusively from academic faculties in medicine and other health professions until 1993. In that year, following the recommendation by the team of independent evaluators the year before, the Foundation extended eligibility for fellowships to all health care professionals, not just academics, including administrators of health maintenance organizations, whether operated for profit or not. But until very recently, attempts to market the program to these organizations hadn't met with much success. That's in part because many of these organizations felt that they couldn't afford to let employees take a year off from work and because many of the potential applicants worried that there wouldn't be a job for them after their year in Washington. And it's in part because candidates from these organizations weren't seen as competitive with the traditional candidates. This has begun to change, however. With the class of 2000–2001, for the first time, half of the Health Policy Fellows came from outside of academic medicine: one from a community health center in Brockport, New York; a second from Anthem Blue Cross and Blue Shield in East Haven, Connecticut; and a third from La Familia Medical Center in Santa Fe, New Mexico.

Whatever the reasons, there has been no significant increase in the pool of applicants from which the six Fellows are chosen each year. That number has averaged about 25 through the years, though for the class of 2001–2002, more than 30 people applied, Lewin said. In fact, one of the questions the Foundation asked an evaluator of the program in 1980 to examine was why the number of applicants was so low. His findings: stipends for the Fellows, $50,000 at the time, were too low; the medical centers, which nominate candidates for fellowships, were complaining that the program wasn't in line with their priorities; and, according to the medical centers, there just weren't enough strong candidates for the fellowships.

The evaluator, Daniel I. Zwick, who at the time was an independent health policy specialist, recommended an increase in the stipends and proposed that the program allow senior faculty members to serve as Fellows. The Foundation accepted both recommendations. Moreover, it took steps to expand the pool of applicants by allowing institutions without medical schools to nominate Fellows and permitting professional schools within academic medical centers to nominate Fellows (previously, academic health centers were limited to a single candidate).

In 2001, the Foundation re-authorized the Health Policy Fellowships Program for an additional three years. It agreed to expand the number of Fellows to ten by the end of the three-year authorization period and to increase the size of the award for each Fellow to $156,000 for the year in Washington plus two follow-up years. The larger grant, according to Lewin, will allow Fellows to remain on Capitol Hill until Congress adjourns, instead of having to leave just as the legislative session approaches its climax. The extra money will also give them some financial flexibility after they finish their fellowships, she added. The program will also put more emphasis on attracting minorities and health professionals with behavioral and social sciences backgrounds, Lewin said.

⟶ Achievements and Failures

Over the years, the fellowship program's methods may have remained the same, but its objectives have been adjusted as evidence accumulated that some of them were unrealistic and that at least one of them was reached with surprising ease. Much of this evidence came from Zwick's 1980 evaluation and from one in 1992 led by David Blumenthal, the chief of the Health Policy Research and Development Unit of Massachusetts General Hospital in Boston and a professor of medicine at Harvard Medical School, who is now the chairman of the Health Policy Fellowships Program's Advisory Board.

1. Preparing for Government Careers

When it established the Health Policy Fellowships Program in 1973, the Foundation's board had stated that one of its purposes was "to provide health professionals who may desire a future career in government an opportunity to prepare for such service."[3] It acted principally on "the perception that leading academicians were frequently tapped for senior health policy positions in the federal government but were ill-prepared to assume these roles."[4] The Foundation officials felt that "an intensive exposure to government early in the careers of these academic health professionals would add enormously to their later effectiveness in governmental roles."[5]

As it turned out, within a few years the Foundation came to see the goal of preparing academics for policy roles in the federal government as unnecessary. Two decades later, however, Blumenthal and his fellow evaluators said that although there was no doubt that the program had failed to achieve that goal, it had succeeded in directing former Fellows "toward involvement in government and community affairs from a base in the private sector." And that was no small accomplishment, they suggested. Their survey of the former Fellows showed that almost one out of five of them had held a federal appointive job, and that most of the rest of them had become active in the health policy arena. More than 56 percent had consulted for a federal program at one time or another, almost 85 percent had stayed in touch with congressional staffs, 63 percent had lobbied Congress, 56 percent had consulted for a federal program, and 38 percent had testified before a congressional committee. Moreover, 58 percent had lobbied state legislatures and 35 percent had advised governors.

That sounds good, but how much of it can properly be attributed to the Health Policy Fellowships Program? Blumenthal and the other evaluators, Gregg S. Meyer and Jennifer N. Edwards, expanded on their survey in a *Health Affairs* essay[6] published in 1994, taking a close look at the differences, if any, between the former Fellows and those who were finalists for fellowships but didn't make the final cut. Their premise was that the two groups were fundamentally alike in most respects: those who selected the Fellows told the evaluators that all of the finalists were "highly qualified."

The survey showed that "significantly more Fellows [than finalists] had participated in one or more academic health policy activities" and that Fellows were likelier than finalists to have participated in several kinds of community and professional activities. These activities included serving in a leadership position or as a health policy adviser in a professional organization, serving as an HMO executive, directing a community health center, and serving on a medical peer review organization. The former Fellows were also likelier than the finalists to be in contact with congressional staffs, to testify or lobby Congress and state legislatures, and to serve in the federal government.

So if the program hasn't succeeded in directing Fellows toward full-time government service, it has managed to point them, as private citizens, in the direction of active involvement in government and community affairs.

2. Influencing Academic Medicine

When the Foundation's staff first began putting together the plan for what became the Health Policy Fellowships Program, academic health centers, or AHCs, "were viewed as the center of the health and health care universe," according to Lewis G. Sandy, the Foundation's executive vice-president, and Richard Reynolds, his predecessor in that post. "The Foundation's staff and board felt that there was an imperfect fit between the mission of AHCs and the needs of the nation," they wrote. "Although not denying the importance and the value of specialty training and practice, the Foundation felt that the declining interest in primary care and the need for a health care workforce that could care for a population's health needs were critical issues not being addressed by AHC leaders." So instead of awarding grants to support biomedical research, the Foundation decided that "more leverage could be gained by fostering the public and community responsibility of AHCs. . . . From that beginning, then, emerged a series of Foundation grants and programs with the aim of influencing academic medicine."[7]

Among these programs was Health Policy Fellowships. Its designers believed that "an intimate exposure to Washington and its ways" would help future deans and chief executive officers of academic medical centers, health professional schools, and teaching hospitals to "develop the skills necessary to interact more constructively and effectively with the federal government."

But the Foundation's ambitious attempt to change the culture of the academic medical centers missed its mark. By 1992, it had become evident that the Fellows were not having the hoped-for impact on their parent institutions. The medical centers, according to the Blumenthal evaluation team, were "embedded in and wedded to a health care system that has defied every major effort at reform over the last 50 years." That is still the case today, according to Blumenthal. "I think their resistance bent but did not break under managed care, and I think that what you're seeing now is the triumph of the counterrevolution," he said in a recent interview. "With the end of managed care as we knew it, reform is still a long way away."

The goal of making academic health centers more socially responsive seemed unattainable by such a small fellowship program. As Sandy and Reynolds concluded, "single agents for change faced difficulties in altering well-entrenched organizational behavior" of the academic centers.[8]

From the Foundation's viewpoint, the biggest problem has been the unwillingness of academic health centers to confront change—or at least the kind of change the Foundation has been pressing for since the early 1970s. The Fellows, after a year in Washington, were changed, "but their old institution was still the same," Steven Schroeder, the president and CEO of The Robert Wood Johnson Foundation, wrote in 1995. As a consequence, he said, the Foundation "changed its expectations about the fellowship's impact on sponsoring institutions."[9]

Over the program's quarter-century of life, a majority of the Fellows have returned, at least initially, to the institutions for which they worked before going to Washington. This was once quite important to the Foundation, whose attempt to influence academic medicine seemed to rely on the Fellows—or at least most of them—returning to the place where they would best be able to effect change. It is less important today, and the goal has largely been set aside.

In fact, the 1992 evaluation recommended that Fellows no longer be "obligated" to return to their sponsoring institutions (though, of course, it was never a legal requirement that they return). Instead, they should be encouraged "to pursue the career option that would best develop their personal potential."

The Foundation board, however, did not accept that recommendation, deciding that it was "too large a shift," Sandy said. "We didn't want to toss the baby out with the bathwater in terms of its academic roots and the idea of a pathway from and then back to academia. Where we came out was with a 'softer' version of that recommendation, which was to be cognizant of the fact that people might not return full time to academia but would find their background applicable in other health policymaking settings."

Subsequently, the nominating procedure was changed to require the sponsoring organization to promise that the nominee would have "an appropriate" position to return to after the fellowship and to outline its plan to use the Fellow's new skills on his or her return. Nevertheless, program director Lewin said, the medical center officer who has made the promise is often gone from the institution, or at least from his or her former position, by the time the Fellow returns, or the institutions "are so strapped or have so many other pressures" that they sometimes can't keep their promises. In any case, Lewin added, those who go somewhere else often improve their job status, so that the move must be considered "a positive, not a negative," for the former Fellows.

But this begs the question that seems to have troubled the Foundation and the evaluators most: Why were the academic health centers reluctant to let their best and brightest participate in the Health Policy Fellowships Program?

For one thing, the academic health centers—all of which include a medical school, at least one other health professional school or program and at least one teaching hospital—were never delighted at the prospect that some of their mid-career faculty members would be trained, in effect, to leave the centers for government service. Zwick, writing in 1982 about his evaluation of the program two years earlier, noted that some of the centers were already worried about the increased risk of losing some of their academic stars.[10] Over time, that fear does not seem to have abated, Lewin said, and "the ownership that academia has felt in this program has declined a little bit because they're not sure everyone is going to return." And as academic medical centers find themselves increasingly in a competitive financial situation, "they can't afford to lose a key health care professional who could be bringing in revenue," said Michael Rothman, the Foundation's senior program officer overseeing the Health Policy Fellowships Program.

Adding to the tension, according to Schroeder, is the fact that what the Fellows learn during their year in Washington "is not mainstream in the lives of academic medical centers," which are primarily interested in basic research and highly specialized health care delivery, not in health policy.

The prospective fellowship candidates, for their part, are worried about what awaits them if they return to the medical centers after a year in Washington. Will their old job be there when they come back? What affect might restructuring, mergers, or strategic alliances have on their prospects for a smooth return? Will their mentors have left in their absence, as happened with David Stevens at Case Western Reserve? Will their absence for a year have cost them opportunities for advancement? And if resources for new programs are scarce at their institution, will the returning Fellows be able to capitalize on what they've learned during their 12 months in Washington?

3. Providing Health Care Expertise to Congress

Ironically, what seemed a lesser objective when the Foundation initiated the Health Policy Fellowships Program has turned out to be one of the program's major successes: making these health professionals available for nine-month assignments at congressional committees in the health field. It is widely agreed that this has worked very well. So a program devised largely to benefit the individual Fellows and to effect change at their institutions has received praise as a tool to assist Congress as it considers health policy legislation.

The program's web site boasts that the Fellows are on the Hill "not as onlookers, but as full-time, working participants," helping to develop legislative proposals, arrange hearings, brief legislators for committee meetings and for floor debates, and working with congressional staffs in House and Senate conferences. During their time in Washington, the Fellows have helped to satisfy the congressional craving for expert medical knowledge and advice. Or so affirm congressional aides who have worked with the Fellows.

The 1992 evaluation found that some congressional aides were initially skeptical about the "amateur" status of the Health Policy Fellows. This was particularly true among majority aides to most of the major committees with health policy jurisdiction, who also insisted that they didn't have the time to train new people every year and were concerned that the Fellows wouldn't always be available and would be gone just as the legislative season reached its climax late in the year. Nevertheless, the evaluators reported, most of these doubters were "generally positive about the program as a whole," and the reluctance of majority aides to sign Fellows up for nine months seems to have diminished recently.

Aides to minority members of the major committees and those who worked on the personal staffs of members of Congress involved in health policy were much more willing to enlist the Fellows on their staffs and much more enthusiastic about their performance. That's at least in part because these legislators are less likely to have sufficient staff assistance and expertise in this area. "The fellowships are good for us and good for them," one such aide told the evaluation team. Another said of the Fellows that they provided "another pair of hands and a good brain." But some agreed with the skeptics that the Fellows were not always available when needed and that the program ended too early in the legislative session.

The Health Policy Fellowships Program was even the source of political controversy during the congressional debate over President Clinton's health care plan in 1993 and 1994. Frank Karel, the Foundation's vice-president for communications, explained that the Foundation organized community meetings to open up the process and let people tell their stories and express their views to Hillary Clinton. "Because of this, and because so many of our grantees were involved in that presidential initiative, hostile critics of the Foundation accused us of partisanship, and were widely quoted," he wrote recently.[11] Foundation executive vice-president Sandy added in a recent interview that the fellowship program was caught up in the "white-hot politics" surrounding the Clinton plan. "We got beat up over the Foundation's role in the planning process and the politicization of health policy," he said.

Lewin agreed that "there was some short-term anger and negative feelings," but, she added, "it blew over very quickly." Almost every year, she said, an article is published "that views the Fellows as agents of the 'liberal' Robert Wood Johnson Foundation and its agenda, but it is never taken seriously." And Paul C. Harrington, who was the majority health policy director for the Senate Health, Education, Labor and Pensions Committee until the Democrats took control of the Senate in June 2001, noted that because the Fellows were working for offices engaged in drafting controversial health legislation in 1993–94, it's understandable that they were caught up in the legislative debate. The program and the Foundation, he said, "were tarred with a brush, unfairly I think, because it didn't reflect an understanding of the role of the Fellowship program." In the years since then, he added, these suspicions have largely been "dispelled, and the Fellows are held in high esteem." After his boss, Senator James M. Jeffords of Vermont (then a Republican), became committee chairman in 1997, he picked a Fellow each year to work for the committee. The committee's new Democratic chairman, Edward M. Kennedy of Massachusetts, has also regularly selected Fellows to work for the panel.

What helped the program weather the small storm, Lewin suggested, was the fact that in its earliest days, it had "gained a unique reputation," and that "to this day, it is still considered the gold standard of health policy fellowships." The program also quite quickly became very valuable to congressional offices, she added, "and many of these offices have come to rely on these people" as sources of expert advice, especially because they have clinical experience.

4. Changing Lives and Promoting Career Development

In 1992, the evaluation team surveyed alumni of the program and found that 81 percent of them agreed with the statement that their fellowship experience had "changed the way I think" and that 60 percent agreed that "it changed my life." Recent anecdotal evidence suggests that those views are still widely held. "It was the most wonderful year of my life," Robert H. Miller, an ophthalmologist, and a member of the class of 1996–97, recalled in an interview. Miller, who returned to Tulane University Medical Center as vice chancellor for clinical affairs after his fellowship and became dean of the University of Nevada School of Medicine in December of 1999, said he didn't doubt that his Washington experience—he worked in the office of Senator John B. Breaux, Democrat of Louisiana—helped him get his current post, which requires intensive courting of state legislators. His fellowship, he added, taught him how the political process—whether in Washington or in the state capital—really works.

The 1992 survey of former Fellows offers statistical support for these examples. The survey found that 80 percent of the Fellows agreed that they were "highly satisfied" with the program, that 98 percent would do it again, and that 99 percent would recommend the program to colleagues. A majority said that the program had helped a lot in achieving their career goals, and more than two-thirds said that it had contributed a lot to their career satisfaction, particularly in the areas of community and government relations and academic administration rather than in academic pursuits such as teaching, researching, and publishing.

Lewin, who has worked closely with each class of Fellows since she became the program's second director, in 1987, said that they have had a chance to learn how Congress really works, how difficult it is for diverse interests to achieve agreement and how democratic the system really is. "The Fellows consider it a life-changing experience," she said.

⁓ Measuring Success

Despite the program's having had to modify its goals over the years and a sense that the program may have been too modest for its ambitious objectives, the Foundation has never balked at renewing it—most recently, in the spring of 2001. "This is an ongoing investment in people, and it's a signature program" for the Foundation, Lewin said. But she quickly added that there may well come a time when something else takes its place.

Measuring the effect even of a program that has a concrete target—reducing the number of children who lack health insurance, say, or improving the long-term care of the elderly—can be a daunting task. Evaluating a program such as the Health Policy Fellowships, whose goals have shifted over time and whose objectives have sometimes been as broad as influencing the nature of academic medicine in the United States, can be almost overwhelming.

"This is the kind of program you shouldn't try to quantify," Schroeder warned. "We're looking for *qualitative* signs," such as the reputation of the Fellows, the nature of their fellowship experience, what they do after it ends. "There's a certain sniff test," he added. "If you're getting people who are good, and if they go on to do good things, then it's probably worth keeping. If you're getting marginal people who don't seem to have much impact on the Hill and don't seem to have much of an impact after their fellowships, then it might not make sense to continue the program."

David Blumenthal, in a recent interview, said that the program's inability to accomplish much in the way of reforming the academic medical centers amounted to the "failure of an unrealistic goal." There continues to be "an enormous gap in culture and understanding between the academic health centers and Washington policymakers," he said. "There are some deans and academic leaders who are quite sophisticated, but it's much more common that they're not." The fellowships program, Blumenthal acknowledged, "has made a modest difference in that regard. There are a small number of deans who are graduates of that program, and they certainly have a deeper understanding of the Washington process."

Certainly the program has made its mark on Capitol Hill, if not in the academic institutions. Though winning praise on the Hill was never part of the program's goals, it might have been shut down long ago if the reviews had been negative.

According to their own testimony, the Fellows have benefited in career terms from the program. Their fellow faculty members have identified them as resources on health policy. And they've maintained their connections with people in Congress and in the executive branch.

Schroeder, in his 1995 article on the program, noted that fellowship programs are expensive (the annual cost has been more than $1 million for a class of six, and will rise to more than $2.5 million as the number of Fellows climbs to ten a year and as the grant to each Fellow increases) and, of necessity, long-term. But in addition to costs, they have "another disadvantage when competing for Foundation support," he acknowledged. They are "relatively invisible" to a foundation's staff and trustees. "The payoffs for the other programs are more immediate. It is easier to judge the quality of research and demonstration programs, the impact of a television documentary or the grandeur of a college library than it is to assess the impact of a fellowship program." Nevertheless, he wrote, The Robert Wood Johnson Foundation supports this and other fellowship programs, "stimulated by the conviction that their impact is enduring and that foundations are almost uniquely positioned to invest in such long-range projects."[12]

So what lessons have been learned about the Health Policy Fellowships Program? Lewin echoes a theme stated by the evaluation team in 1992: that the program needs to be more aggressively marketed. She acknowledged that to some former Fellows, it's an exclusive club, and "once you advertise it, it loses some of its appeal."

The evaluators had suggested marketing the program to faculty below the top level instead of relying on the institutions to act as intermediaries. But while this is clearly a way to increase the pool of applicants, it could be a risky step. Sandy, in an interview, pointed out that "the institutional sponsorship of the Fellows is part of the brand identity of the program within Washington," and said that if the fellows come without that sponsorship, "that may dilute the brand equity in the whole fellowship" and might even suggest that the Fellows have individual political agendas. That's something the Foundation would want to avoid, he said.

As to the role that the Fellows play after leaving Washington, the evaluators observed almost a decade ago that "affecting the career development of its alumni is, in fact, the most fundamental purpose of any fellowship program." They added, "If fellows are to become agents of change, they must first be changed themselves."

Blumenthal, who continues to pay close attention to the program as the chairman of its Advisory Board, was asked recently if, indeed, former Fellows had become "agents of change." His response: "I think they've tried to function as agents of change. I think it's unrealistic to expect 150-odd people to change a health care system of a trillion and a half dollars."

What's in the offing, then, for this program after more than a quarter of a century?

The Foundation has come to terms with the fact that the Health Policy Fellowships Program will never achieve the ambitious goals originally set for it: preparing health professionals for careers in government and changing the face of academic medicine in America. That, as it turned out, was too much of a reach for such a relatively modest program. Yet the program has altered the professional careers of the Fellows and is perceived in Washington as valuable. It continues to be one of what the Foundation calls its "core programs." Like other core programs, such as the Clinical Scholars Program, it has been around a long time. So, despite some shortfalls in reaching all of its goals and despite its high cost, it has become part of the institutional fabric of the Foundation and is likely to remain part of that fabric for some years to come.

Notes

1. J. Shecter, "Medical Dean Turned Senate Aide," *The Chronicle of Higher Education*, May 24, 1996.
2. The Institute of Medicine and Massachusetts General Hospital, *National Program Report*, unpublished report to The Robert Wood Johnson Foundation, February 1999, p. 4.
3. D. Blumenthal, G. S. Meyer, and J. N. Edwards, *The Robert Wood Johnson Foundation Health Policy Fellowship: an Evaluation*, unpublished report to The Robert Wood Johnson Foundation, December, 1992, pp. 3–4.
4. Ibid, p. 3.
5. Ibid, p. 3.
6. G. S. Meyer, J. N. Edwards, D. Blumenthal, "Experience of the Robert Wood Johnson Foundation Health Policy Fellowship," *Health Affairs*, 1994, volume 13, number 2, pp. 264–270.
7. L. G. Sandy and R. Reynolds, "Influencing Academic Health Centers: The Robert Wood Johnson Foundation Experience," *To Improve Health and*

Health Care, 1998–1999, The Robert Wood Johnson Foundation Anthology (San Francisco: Jossey-Bass, 1998), pp. 81–99.

8. Ibid.

9. Institute of Medicine Council, "The Institute of Medicine's Review of the Health Policy Fellowships Program," in *For the Public Good: Highlights from the Institute of Medicine, 1970–1995* (Washington, D.C.: National Academy Press, 1995).

10. D. I. Zwick, "Evaluation of the Robert Wood Johnson Health Policy Fellowship Program: A Synopsis," in *Journal of Health Politics, Policy and Law,* 1982, volume 6, number 4.

11. F. Karel, "'Getting the Word Out': A Foundation Memoir and Personal Journey," *To Improve Health and Health Care 2001: The Robert Wood Johnson Foundation Anthology* (San Francisco: Jossey-Bass, 2001), pp. 39–40.

12. Institute of Medicine Council, "The Institute of Medicine's Review of the Health Policy Fellowships Program," in *For the Public Good: Highlights from the Institute of Medicine,* 1970–1995 (Washington, D.C.: National Academy Press, 1995).

A Closer Look

CHAPTER SEVEN

⟶ Recovery High School

Digby Diehl

Editors' Introduction

Alternative schools emerged in the 1960s as a way of offering programs designed to meet the educational and therapeutic needs of troubled youngsters who were not succeeding in the public school system. They were seen by their advocates as an answer to juvenile crime and delinquency, a means of reducing school violence, and a way of increasing educational effectiveness.

In this chapter, best-selling author Digby Diehl tells the story of Recovery High in Albuquerque, New Mexico, an alternative school for substance-abusing adolescents. It is a story that, although focused on an individual school, raises troubling issues of great importance for our society. Are alternative schools an effective way to meet the therapeutic and educational needs of young people with substance abuse problems? What is a fair way to allocate funds between meeting the normal educational needs of most children and the extended and more costly needs of those with special disorders? Who should bear the cost of treating and educating substance-abusing children—the educational, justice, health, or social service system, or some other system?

The grant to the Albuquerque Public School District was an unusual one for The Robert Wood Johnson Foundation in a number of ways. The Foundation does very little with schools, since education is not one of its priorities. It is also rare to receive a grant request from a group of concerned parents rather than an established organization. Recovery High does, however, demonstrate the importance to the Foundation of ad hoc grants, those based on unsolicited requests sent by individuals. This grant-making mechanism allows the Foundation to support creative ideas from people who want to make a difference, and enables the Foundation's staff to learn about potential emerging areas of grantmaking.

Thanks to Recovery High, I have been sober for seven years. The school is where I got the strength and confidence I needed, because when I went in I had no self-esteem. These people showed that they cared for me, that they were there for me no matter what. Walking out of that school was probably the hardest thing I ever had to do.

> Andrea Blaine
> Former Student
> Recovery High

Recovery High was known as a safe place, a drug-free place, a therapeutic place. Clinically, it was working. Politically, it was a disaster.

> Buzz Biernacki
> Former President
> Recovery High Board

Recovery High was ignored as a resource for the very school system it was intended to serve. The system had nothing but contempt for us. No matter how hard we tried, no matter what processes we went through to reach out, they simply wouldn't refer students to us.

> Michael Hays
> Former History/English Teacher
> Recovery High

There's a lot of moral stuff around substance abuse that people can't let go of; they don't understand it's a disease. They see it as something morally wrong—which made us controversial.

> Jan Hayes
> Former Principal
> Recovery High

I never had an interest in Recovery High School, so it's the only school I haven't visited. I never saw it as permanent. I don't think of it as a school, more like a therapy institution.

Board Member
Albuquerque Board of Education[1]

I truly believe that the basis for most of the resistance to Recovery High was a deep-seated feeling that these children should not be seen and not be heard. That attitude was reflected by the society, by the school district, by the families, by individuals. Substance abuse was perceived as a shameful fault, not as a medical or psychological problem. These children were regarded as inferior. On a personal level, I was shocked that parents and educators were not flocking to the doors of Recovery High to bring us kids. I saw those kids every night in the Emergency Room.

Robert Gougelet
Emergency Room Physician and
Former Recovery High Project Liaison

There were people saying, "Those kids aren't worth it. We're spending money on kids that aren't worth a damn, and the good kids are getting short-changed." To many people, Recovery High was like a wart.

Jack Bobroff
Former Superintendent
Albuquerque Public Schools

Recovery High School was an innovative alternative school in Albuquerque, New Mexico, for adolescents who were dependent on drugs and alcohol. The school integrated educational, therapeutic, and medical services. Funded primarily by The Robert Wood Johnson Foundation and supported, with increasing reluctance, by the Albuquerque Public Schools Board, it was in operation from February, 1992, to May, 1995. The quotations represent the dichotomy of attitudes within the community about Recovery High. Ultimately, this polarization over the value of the school, coupled with the expense of running it, proved to be its undoing.

—— Origins

Recovery High originated with one man. Lou Sadler was a determined Albuquerque father whose son was a substance abuser. Like many parents faced with this problem, Sadler found it difficult to get his child the help he needed. At the time, teenage substance abusers were like pinballs in a particularly merciless arcade game, forcefully colliding with various posts and pillars in the social fabric—the schools, the cops, the courts, their families, inpatient facilities, outpatient facilities, detention facilities—only to ricochet back and forth among them because no single institution could give them the comprehensive help they needed. Teenage substance abusers were everyone's problem but no one's responsibility.

The Albuquerque public school system is one of the largest in the country, in terms of both geography and population. Covering a landscape the size of Rhode Island, with 120 schools and 85,000 students, the district also lies at the crossroads of two major drug pipelines—Interstate 25, by which drugs come north from Mexico, and Interstate 40, which links California ports of entry with Arizona, New Mexico, Texas, and the south. Illegal drugs flowing through Albuquerque include powder cocaine and crack cocaine, marijuana, black-tar heroin, and methamphetamine. (Much of the methamphetamine is locally manufactured.) In 1990, the Albuquerque area was included in a federally designated High Intensity Drug Trafficking Area. According to the Office of National Drug Control Policy, "Gangs facilitate much of the drug distribution that occurs at street level and are responsible for much of the drug-related violence in the region."[2]

In 1990, the rate of teenage deaths by accident, homicide, and suicide in New Mexico was 70 percent higher than the national average.[3] Some 2,000 Albuquerque public school students were suspended for substance abuse every year, and more than 500 middle-school and upper-school students in the Albuquerque school system were receiving treatment for chemical dependency. The New Mexico Boys and Girls Schools, which are juvenile-correction facilities, were admitting more than 800 juveniles annually, most of whom were from the Albuquerque area.[4]

An unknown number left the system before getting treatment, but even for kids who got professional help, relapses into drug use were the norm, not the exception.[5] Most teenagers recovering from alcohol or chemical dependency who returned home were shunned by straight students once they reentered school, and they were not strong enough emotionally to rebuff overtures from substance-abusing former friends. Sadler's own son relapsed repeatedly, and was in and out of a series of conventional inpatient treatment centers. "Kids who spend four weeks in those places dry out and come home sober, but only because they've been under lock and key for a month," Sadler says. "I got pretty frustrated with facilities that turn out thirty-day wonders. They all claimed a low recidivism rate, but it never worked out that way. My son eventually got into trouble with the law, so I was finally able to get him into a very tough long-term treatment program in Texas that was successful. From that experience, I realized that recovery had to be a long-term process for a child—for anybody."

Helping his son become clean and sober did little to elevate Sadler's opinion of the way the Albuquerque public school system handled recovering substance abusers. In fact, the approach was inconsistent. Some students who had left school to participate in rehab programs were told upon trying to return to class that they had been dropped from the rolls for excessive absenteeism. Others, Sadler's son among them, were dumped back into the same classes they had left, with little or no effort made to cover the material they had missed. "My son ended up being out of school for three months, and they *still* graduated him," says Sadler, who is a no-nonsense builder-contractor. "I thought that was ignorant and bad and stupid."

With a reputation for being plainspoken and assertive if not downright confrontational, Sadler closed his contracting business and threw himself full force into the problem, becoming a member of New Mexico Governor Garrey Carruthers' Substance Abuse Advisory Council, and Albuquerque Mayor Ken Schultz's Kitchen Cabinet. With a group of other individuals, he founded Parents Against Drugs, a private, nonprofit organization of parents, community activists, and treatment professionals, in 1987. Led by Sadler, Parents Against Drugs set out to develop a better way to help teenagers who were abusing drugs and alcohol. "I wanted to come up with something that would enable kids to stay sober, and allow them to continue their education," Sadler says.

Using political connections and the media effectively, he and Parents Against Drugs mobilized governmental machinery to start an alternative educational facility for recovering substance abusers—in effect, a magnet school for kids who were newly sober. In 1989, Parents Against Drugs was instrumental in pushing a resolution through the New Mexico legislature "requesting a study of the feasibility of creating an alternative education magnet school for students with substance abuse problems."[6] The Albuquerque City Council and the Albuquerque Public Schools Board both endorsed the concept, but only with the reservation that the school be "built and operated through funds provided entirely by private foundations and federal and state government."[7] The indefatigable Sadler then spearheaded a drive to find funding for the school, and wrote to The Robert Wood Johnson Foundation.

"I received a letter from Parents Against Drugs," recalls Paul Jellinek, a vice-president of The Robert Wood Johnson Foundation. "Initially, the group wanted a truckload of money to build a new school; I advised them to go after a small planning grant that would help them refine their model of how an alternative education facility would function."

As a result, the Foundation gave Parents Against Drugs $75,000 to flesh out the concept. Jellinek also made another crucial recommendation. "I told them that once they'd developed a plan for a school, a major organization would have to take responsibility for it," he says. "There was no way that The Robert Wood Johnson Foundation could give a large grant to what was essentially an informal group of parents. My own instincts were that the best way to do this was through the Albuquerque public school system, so that whatever school was developed was integrated into the broader system."

⸺ The Model

The school was originally conceived as a transitional facility, a "halfway school" for young people who had successfully completed a course of treatment for substance abuse. These were to be "moderately troubled adolescents whose primary need was to be isolated from the drug culture of their schools."[8]

The alternative school was established to "provide a program of adolescent substance abuse, recovery, and relapse prevention within a supportive educational setting. . . . The goal was to enable adolescents to return to the regular school system with the support and skills necessary to remain abstinent."[9] Students were expected to spend six months to a year at this way station before returning to a conventional high school. To minimize contact with drug-using old friends, this was not, in most cases, expected to be the school they had left. As a defense against ostracism in their new environment, the plan called for "graduates" to be mainstreamed out not singly but in small groups, so that they could form their own peer support networks at their new school.

With "aftercare" or reentry kids as the primary target population, the Parents Against Drugs proposal anticipated being able to serve up to 200 students at a time. Before the school opened, however, the proposal was modified to include students who had not had any formal treatment. The change was made to enable the school to become a resource for the large number of teenagers in Albuquerque who were uninsured (estimated to be about 30 percent of the school population),[10] and who thus had no other access to substance abuse treatment. "We wanted this school to be open for anybody who really needed it," says Robert Gougelet, a University of New Mexico professor of emergency medicine and physician who was involved in setting up the program.

During the planning phase, Sadler and others researched the handful of educational facilities in different parts of the country that also tried to combine academics with therapy for teenage substance abusers.[11] With the experience of these other schools incorporated into the model, the alternative school began to take shape.

The Parents Against Drugs proposal defined three goals for the program: (1) maintenance of sobriety; (2) improvement of family relationships and support; and (3) educational success in a program that integrated recovery skills with education.[12] Progress toward these goals was monitored by Susan Leonard Thaler and Paul Moberg of the University of Wisconsin's Center for Health Policy and Program Evaluation, who were retained by The Robert Wood Johnson Foundation.

The therapeutic model chosen for the school was that of a community or milieu in which "teachers, clinicians, support staff, students, and the students' families are all involved in the development of a recovery process for the student, focused around the 12 Steps of Alcoholics Anonymous."[13] The idea was to create a positive environment within the school that would support a comprehensive change in both attitude and behavior. The community itself was to function as the primary therapist, and within it, anything and everything was therapeutic. Key components included art therapy and experiential or wilderness training, with a ropes course and other outdoor activities. The involvement of family members in the recovery process was believed to be critical. Although the school planned to use the standard curriculum of the Albuquerque public school system, by design there was to be no real division between academics and therapy.

In response to the 300-page proposal submitted by Parents Against Drugs, in April of 1991 The Robert Wood Johnson Foundation awarded an $812,000 implementation grant to the Albuquerque Public School District to get the school up and running. Four months later, the school board grudgingly appropriated $267,000 in matching seed money for the alternative school, with the proviso that the board would support the facility for only a two-year period.

—ᐧᐧᐧ— Start-Up

The original organization chart for the school called for a project director at the head, a "big picture" individual who would be responsible not only for coordinating the program but also for dealing with external bureaucracies, including state and local governmental authorities and the school system itself. The most important responsibility of the project director was to raise funds, in order to establish the long-term financial security of the school. This fund-raising assignment would play a decisive part in the future of Recovery High, since neither The Robert Wood Johnson Foundation nor the Albuquerque school board intended to continue funding the project over the long term.

Having brought the concept this far, Lou Sadler was the most likely candidate to become project director, and on July 25, 1991, he signed a contract with the Albuquerque Public School District to head the school. The opening date was set for October 15 of that year. Three professionals were to handle the day-to-day running of the school under Sadler's direction: a full-time principal responsible for academics and daily administration; a full-time intervention director to oversee the therapy program; and a part-time medical director to deal with the children's health needs.

On September 3, Jan Hayes, an external candidate for the position, was hired as principal. Three days later, and just six weeks before the projected opening day, the school board canceled its contract with Sadler for having misrepresented his educational qualifications on his résumé. His abrupt departure delayed the opening of the school by four months, and left Jan Hayes as the de facto head of the entire school, not just the educational component.[14]

Jack Bobroff, who was then superintendent of schools and a supporter of the concept, fired Sadler at the direction of the board of education. The circumstances were curious. "One of our board members got an anonymous telephone call saying that Lou Sadler didn't have a college degree," Bobroff says. "In soliciting applications for project director, we hadn't asked for one, but the board found it unacceptable that a person would not tell the truth on his résumé, and on that basis Lou was terminated. In many ways, that contributed greatly to the downfall of the program. With his tenacity and his fervor, Lou had been a great moving force, and that was lost. Jan Hayes did a good job dealing with the kids and running the program, but she had her hands full with the internal workings of the school. She didn't have time to pursue fundraising."

Sadler still regrets his misstep. "I attended the University of Maryland, but never graduated," he says. "On my résumé, I said I'd gotten a degree. I gave the board a reason to get rid of me, and that was bad. Because they never replaced me, even though they had the money, they lost the opportunity to really go ahead and create funding and long-term programs for the school."

Sadler's fiery exit made it inevitable that the school would be born in a barrage of controversy and bad press.[15] There was even a flap about what to call it. Some within the district argued strongly for an innocuous Southwestern name—Mariposa (butterfly) was a leading contender. In the end, it was the students themselves who spoke up for the truth-in-packaging approach, and dubbed the school Recovery High. It finally opened its doors at 2700 Yale SE on February 18, 1992, with a staff of 12 and a student body of 3.[16]

~~~ Theory Meets Reality

Although Sadler and Parents Against Drugs had been conscientious in developing the plan for the school, from the first day Recovery High never functioned according to the original model. The low enrollment indicated more than just the school's start-up woes; it reflected a genuine and deep-seated reluctance on the part of other members of the Albuquerque public school system community to refer students to Recovery High. Fewer than a quarter of all Recovery High students were referred by a school counselor or an administrator.[17] "We were astonished by some of the responses we got, especially from principals," says Michael Hays, who taught English and history at Recovery High. "Principals told us, 'We don't have a drug problem in our school'—but I don't know of a school that doesn't have one."

Although denial was undoubtedly a major factor, a lot of the problem at the beginning boiled down to dollars and cents. By law, every school district in New Mexico gets its funding from the state, and under what is known as the New Mexico equalization formula, the school district distributes to each school its fair share based on its enrolled population. One date each October is designated as school Census Day, when the school system literally counts heads and divvies up the budget accordingly. This simple formula produced some unintended consequences for the new school. Former Recovery High Board President Buzz Biernacki knew how the math was done: "At budget time, if your school had 100 kids, you got 100 slices of the pie. But if you only had 90 kids because Recovery High had your 10 others, you got ten slices less of the pie. So if you were a school principal, you weren't about to fess up to any substance abuse problem until after that October cutoff date."

After the October census, however, principals of mainstream schools had an incentive to purge substance-abusing students. Not only were they ridding their school of "troublemakers," but they also got to keep the money. Whether students transferred to Recovery High, were expelled, or simply dropped out, their per capita allocations were retained by the school of record. In 1992, the Albuquerque Public School District was in a budget crunch; arts programs were being gutted, and even sports were being pruned back. Not surprisingly, the principals were zealously protective of any found money. "The high school principals were totally nonsupportive prior to the October cutoff," Biernacki recalls. "But on October 14 or whatever the mystery date was, we'd get the call: 'For God's sake, send some counselors over here and pick up these kids!'"

This was not the referral process the staff had envisioned; "picking up" students in response to an appeal from an exasperated principal was inimical to the Recovery High program. "We had our own strict criteria, which wouldn't allow kids in who were just being tossed at us," says Michael Hays. "Students had to come to the school of their own volition. There had to be a clear, desperate commitment on the part of the child entering the program. We did not accept students who said they didn't want to be here." In the first semester of the school's existence, 53 placement interviews were conducted, resulting in 31 enrollments. Eight of those not admitted were denied because of "excessive medications, gang involvement, history of violent behavior, or lack of willingness to commit to recovery." The fourteen others were simply not interested in attending Recovery High.[18]

In the earliest days of Recovery High, the first task of the staff was to structure the program. It developed a point and level system to evaluate student progress. All students entered the school at Level 1, and accumulated points to move up to Levels 2 and 3. Points were awarded hourly on a scale of 1 to 4 for staying on task, interaction with others, positive risk-taking, willingness to accept personal responsibility, and other hallmarks of recovery. On any given school day, it was theoretically possible for a student to accumulate 200 points. In practice, a 150-point day was about average, a 180-point day was outstanding, and a 100- to 120-point day was all too common.

Within the milieu of the school, Level 1s were designated as observers, with limited privileges and limited responsibilities. They were expected to become familiar with the way the school functioned by watching other members of the community (both staff members and more advanced students), and were not permitted to voice an opinion or to vote at community meetings. Limiting the privileges of Level 1s not only curtailed their propensity to act out but also reinforced the concept that they were at the bottom of the pecking order. To move up to Level 2, they needed to earn 700 points for two consecutive weeks.

Level 2s were designated as members of the community, participated in discussions, and had voting privileges. Level 3s were the leaders of the student body, and had a range of privileges that approached that of students in a conventional high school, including the right to leave the campus for lunch. To progress to Level 3, Level 2s had to show two consecutive 800-point weeks. All promotions of Level 1 and 2 students had to be presented to the community by a Level 3 sponsor and endorsed by the group.

～ Inside Recovery High

For faculty and staff members, the school day began with a coordination meeting at 7:30 a.m. to discuss student progress or particular issues that had arisen. The school functioned with pairs of counselors and teachers, who worked together as a primary care team and dealt with a caseload of ten to fifteen adolescents. The students arrived at 8:00 a.m. and met with their primary care team at the opening bell for goal-setting (they met again at 4:30 p.m. for an end-of-the-day review). At goal setting, students wrote down their objectives for the day on their point sheets, which they carried around with them to each class and activity.

After one class period, the entire school—students, teachers, counselors, principal, secretary, and janitor—convened for a community meeting. Each day, Level 3 students chose one of their own as moderator for the meeting. After a moment of silence, the first question asked by the moderator was always the same: "Does anyone have anything to say about their recovery, or a confrontation to make?"

Attendance at the community meeting was mandatory—as were openness and honesty. There were no secrets at Recovery High. Any student who had relapsed was expected to confess it at the meeting—and thereafter face a cross-examination by the group. Failure to come forward carried a far greater risk—if other members of the community knew of or suspected another's relapse, they were duty-bound to declare their suspicion and confront the individual. "Because community meetings were intrinsic to milieu therapy, they were very powerful, especially when students confronted one another," Michael Hays says.

Whether a relapse was confessed or was revealed by confrontation, the fate of relapsers was in the hands of the community. Expulsion was not automatic, but a drop back to Level 1 was a given. Counselors expected relapses as part of the recovery process, especially for new arrivals; from their perspective, the more important question was what happened next. Relapsing students who acknowledged using drugs but recommitted to the program were offered the support of the community. Those who placed the blame on someone other than themselves, or denied drug use when confronted with proof, found themselves on the brink of expulsion.

"Monday was always interesting, because you'd wonder who'd relapsed over the weekend," principal Jan Hayes says. "They'd come to see me in my office, and I could always tell as soon as they came through that front door, because they'd act different. We did have our share of kids who relapsed, but generally we were able to get them back into recovery. One of the biggest problems our students had was learning how to say, 'I did that'—to be honest and to take responsibility for their actions. If a kid voluntarily came forward without somebody else telling on him, he was in a lot better shape."

Some students who had difficulty with authority figures found it easier to admit a relapse to a support staff member or another student. "When I was a Level 3, I had kids coming to me crying and telling me what happened because they didn't know how to tell the group," Elena Ortiz, a former student, recalls. "We would talk about it together, and that made it easier for them. After you've told one person first, it isn't so scary to tell twenty people."

The secretary and the janitor became key figures in Recovery High. "If kids acted out, a lot of times the consequence was to go help Joe clean toilets," Jan Hayes says. "They'd begin to talk and develop a relationship with him. A lot of students got really close to him, and we got a great deal of information that way that was helpful. Barbara Romero, our secretary, was always there early, so she saw them coming in."

"My role was more like the mother figure," Romero says. "The girls, especially, would come to me in my office when they just needed someone to talk to." The fact that support staff members functioned as a sounding board for students was encouraged by Hayes. "We always told the students, 'You can talk to anybody, and everybody on this staff is equally important. If Barbara or Joe is who you're comfortable talking with, fine, but they're not going to keep a secret if it's something that's going to impinge upon your recovery.'"

Counselors made constructive use of relapses when they did occur. Within the milieu, every crisis was seen as an opportunity for students to take responsibility for their own actions and to trust the community to be there for them in support of their efforts at recovery.

Learning to be accountable for yourself and learning to trust the community safety net were skills that were enhanced by experiential or wilderness therapy. These Outward Bound-style outings challenged students to undertake a frightening or unfamiliar activity—such as rock climbing or cave exploration—in order to experience the personal growth and increased self-esteem that came from successful completion of what had first seemed impossible. Upon occasion, they also provided a painful lesson in the need to follow instructions.

"There was one girl named Tita, who was a tiny, Barbie-doll thing," Jan Hayes says with a smile. "She always had these wonderful clothes and high-heeled fancy shoes. The day before the outing, two of us sat her down and said, 'Now you want to be sure and dress warmly. You need to wear long pants, shoes, and socks.' Sure enough, she shows up in a pair of shorts and strappy sandals, and she's thinking she won't have to go. We just packed her off and sent her right up the mountainside with everyone else. When she started to complain, I said, 'Honey, by the time you come back down, you're gonna have blisters on your little feet, but it's your fault you've got on sandals. You'll have to make it to the top like the rest.'"

To build trust and reinforce the concept of community, counselors and teachers had to be willing to do everything the students did. It was important that all members of the community conquer their fears and participate in these outings—especially staff members. A high ropes course was also part of the Recovery High program, and many staff members were nervous about traversing ropes and cables two stories off the ground. "For a lot of our kids, this was the first time they had adults they could trust," Jan Hayes says. "It was important that we were all positive role models. We wanted to show them that we really cared for them and wanted them to succeed. I thought I wouldn't be able to cross those ropes, but I did."

"Talk about trust and self-esteem—the biggest problem these kids had in six hours up there was holding hands," says Al Benalli, a counselor. "We were up twenty feet in the air on the cable, and they were reluctant to hold hands. They were hanging on to each other's jackets and pants and all that kind of stuff, and I said, 'Well, what about the hands?' They asked me, 'Wasn't it ever hard for you?' I said, 'Yes, but when I was in Vietnam, you'd get out there in the fog and muck and you can't see where you're going. You can't see your hand in front of your face because it's raining, so you hold hands and you can feel the other person. And when you're up there twenty feet in the air, you need that kind of support from somebody else.'"

"When any adventure was over, the group reflected on what was difficult for each member," former teacher Michael Hays recalls. "The adventure then became a compelling metaphor for some aspect of each participant's life as we explored what inhibited, frightened, confused, and motivated us."[19]

Counselors and teachers at Recovery High were addressed by their first names, and were subject to the same code of behavior as the students—a concept that extended to random drug screenings by urinalysis, or UA. What was known within the community as a "dirty UA" was another means by which relapsers were unmasked.[20] Kids who tried to con their way out after testing positive found their bluff called immediately. "Often kids with a dirty UA would deny they did anything," Barbara Romero recalls. "They'd claim that the lab made a mistake. When that happened, we'd send them over there and say, 'O.K., go talk to the guy who runs the lab. We'll get them to do a confirmation on this.'"

"When UAs were given to teachers and counselors, to emphasize the community part, the adolescents got to pick which staff members took the test," counselor Al Sanchez says. "We all had to stay clean." The counselors who became known as 'the two Als'—Sanchez and Benalli—were open about the fact that they are former substance abusers who became sober through the 12-Step Alcoholics Anonymous program; their willingness to undergo random testing not only reinforced students' faith in the program but also underscored the crucial concept that recovery is a lifelong process.

All students participated daily in what was known as "step study"—class time devoted to discussion of the tenets of AA. "It was actively integrated into the language and treatment of the school," Michael Hays says.

Parent involvement was an essential part of the Recovery High program. Parents met with Recovery High staff members once a week. "They had to be educated, too," Jan Hayes says. "They had to learn that this is a disease. They thought we'd be able to get their kids to stop, and that it wouldn't make any difference if they had a refrigerator full of beer. The attitude was 'Why shouldn't I be able to drink? He's got the problem. I don't.' What did we find out? We found out that mom or dad is an alcoholic. Most of these children came from families where drugs and alcohol were a normal part of their lives."

—— A Very Different Student

The school slowly began to attract more students, but it was recognized early on that the goal of having 200 recovering adolescents was unattainable; the objective was halved to a target population of 100, but to the staff members that number was still too high.

In practice, the school usually functioned with 60 students or fewer, and even at that size the arrival of new Level 1 students played havoc with the school's sense of community. Maintaining the integrity of the community or the milieu was crucial to the functioning of Recovery High. For the milieu to be stable, a certain proportion of Level 2 and especially Level 3 students was essential. Without the leadership of students deeply committed to recovery, the milieu broke down; staff members would lead community discussions and make decisions—and thus the milieu would become far more authoritarian.

For this reason, an influx of new students was often traumatic. "When referrals finally came, each new arrival could have such an overpowering effect on the school that the thought of more students nearly caused the faculty to despair," Michael Hays says. "When we got in some very hard kids, it would take weeks to get things rebalanced. They would come in by twos and fours, and it was a while before we could even try to integrate them into the milieu. When the milieu stabilized, we could admit more, again hoping that we could withstand the manipulative, histrionic, or antisocial behavior that arrived with each new student. When we reached an enrollment of approximately 70, we found ourselves nearly overrun."

Many referrals came from the criminal justice system; often these were adolescents who had been given the choice between enrollment at Recovery High and incarceration. Most of the student body had had one or more run-ins with the law. More than half had spent time in a juvenile detention center; almost half had been arrested for a felony. Fifty-four percent were involved with the juvenile justice system at the time they entered Recovery High. Forty percent admitted to active gang membership or affiliation,[21] but staff members confirmed a much more extensive degree of gang involvement.

Other referrals came from treatment facilities. Many students had been in residence at inpatient treatment facilities, and had been discharged—not because they were in recovery but because their length of stay had exhausted their insurance benefits. Virtually all teenagers who entered Recovery High arrived with a far more tenuous hold on sobriety than had been anticipated. Many arrived with no recovery experience whatever, only their good intentions—and often that sincerity was enough for them to be admitted to the program, no matter what else was wrong with them.

And there was plenty wrong with them. Ethnically, the students at Recovery High resembled the demographic cross-section of the

Albuquerque population,[22] but that was the only normal thing about them. "From opening to closing, Recovery High School served a considerably more acute pre-recovery teen, with little or no (mostly "no") prior experience with recovery/sobriety. . . . Students demonstrated a multiplicity of behavioral, mental, and physical issues common to adolescents with serious histories of chemical abuse. These students also arrived with serious family and psychological problems that predated chemical use," Al Sanchez wrote.[23] As tabulated by the Recovery High counseling staff, the litany of psychiatric and social problems experienced by these children is astounding:

- 100% had committed a delinquent act

- 100% were multiple substance abusers

- 76% had been suspended or expelled from school

- 48% had dropped out of school

- 60% had witnessed a violent crime

- 34% had been victims of a violent crime

- 53% reported a history of family violence

- 48% had been physically abused

- 60% had committed a violent act

- 80% had engaged in a violent act with others

- 20% owned a gun

- 44% had dealt drugs

- 60% had engaged in self-mutilation[24]

Half of the students at Recovery High were female. A third of them had been victims of sexual abuse as children; just over half of those were incest victims. All incoming Recovery High students were interviewed about what their lives had been like recently. As documented by the evaluators Moberg and Thaler,[25] their experiences during just the year before their enrollment were harrowing:

- 57% reported a family member abusing alcohol or drugs

- 42% had been kicked out of their homes

- 11% reported a teenage pregnancy (self or partner)
- 62% of the girls had been victims of sexual assault
- 42% of the girls had attempted suicide

All of them came to the school fragile, and most incoming adolescents were afflicted not only by addictive behavior but also by another diagnosable psychiatric disorder. Fully eighty-four percent met criteria for clinical depression.[26] A third of arriving female students and a quarter of arriving male students were suicidal at the time of enrollment.

The extent and the severity of the students' psychological problems also had physical manifestations. At the outset, medical care was given equal emphasis with therapy and academics at Recovery High.[27] A small health clinic was part of the original plan. Robert Gougelet, a physician, drew upon his resources at the University of New Mexico and helped arrange for the clinic to be staffed by a full-time nurse practitioner and a part-time emergency pediatrician. "We had a lot of pregnancy tests, and a lot of education around sexually transmitted diseases," he says. "Because their families hadn't had them go to doctors for ages, kids also came in with all kinds of disorders they weren't aware of—biggies like diabetes and hepatitis."

"They weren't eating regularly; there were a lot of nutrition issues," Jan Hayes adds. "We fed them lunch every day, and it was probably the only meal some of them had." Almost fifty percent of the students (and almost two-thirds of the girls) exhibited signs of an eating disorder.

A formidable array of physical and psychosocial baggage put the students of Recovery High off the chart on any measurement scale of "at risk" youth. "The drugs and alcohol were the least of their problems," Jan Hayes says. "They were the only means by which these kids could medicate their pain."

—⁓— Confluence and Curriculum

It was inevitable that Recovery High students would have significant academic problems, but the faculty members had not anticipated how dysfunctional their students would be in the classroom. About a third of the students who entered in the first year of the program were identified as having a handicap that impeded them academically (learning disability, emotional disability, behavior disorder, attention deficit disorder—a few students were in fact illiterate),[28] and a special-education teacher was eventually added to the staff. Virtually all the students were below grade level, regardless of handicap.

Classes were taught by subject matter, but within each classroom the students were a mixed bag of ages, abilities, IQs, and attention spans—not to mention levels of recovery. Some were fresh from middle school; others were old enough to have already graduated. Of necessity, faculty members resorted to a tutorial approach. Students were handed packets of material, and assignments were designed according to their level of ability.

From time to time, however, teachers were able to find some unlikely common ground for group activity. "We read *A Midsummer Night's Dream,*" Michael Hays recalls. "We sat around a table—hardcore junkies, gang-bangers, skater-punks. . . taking parts and reading Shakespeare together. Once the kids became accustomed to the language, they started laughing spontaneously at some of the things that happened."

Because school had historically been a negative experience for most Recovery High students, the classroom environment often brought out a host of undesirable behavior, often at unpredictable moments. Teachers never knew when a disruption would occur that might require their intervention.

"There was a lot of acting out, a lot of verbal abuse," counselor Al Benalli says. "The kids seemed to think when they used inappropriate language that they might threaten us. I always told them that the only people I was afraid of were adult males who were intoxicated. When you're working with adolescents who've been involved with alcohol and drugs, you have to expect them to be restless, irritable, and discontented. In order to be successful with them, you need to understand that from the first time they used until the time that they got into recovery, their emotional development is arrested. You might have a 16-year-old who is acting like an eight-year-old, but if you're knowledgeable about substance abuse, you can understand that's just natural. The kid stopped growing up when he started using."

"Some of our kids had started using at the age of 8, 9, or 10," Jan Hayes says. "They were so young that they hadn't been habilitated, let alone rehabilitated." The issue was how to find the best way to help them catch up with their peers, both emotionally and academically. The term "confluence" was used to describe the integration of therapy with the academic curriculum. In English class, Michael

Hays assigned students the task of writing the autobiography of their addiction. In keeping with Step 1 of the AA program ("We admit we are powerless over alcohol and that our lives have become unmanageable"), he asked them to describe the moment at which they realized that their lives had become unmanageable. "Kids were writing incredible stuff," he recalls. "I remember a girl who began her story by saying, 'I woke up on somebody's lawn. The sun was hot, and a dog was licking my face.' She'd never written a paper before in her life."

"The children had standard English courses; they were still expected to read the literature and know grammar, but we found that we had to do a lot of high-interest activity-oriented things," Jan Hayes says. Faculty and counselors devised creative ways to blend other academic disciplines with the therapy program. One of the most popular techniques was "excursion class." For civics, students went to the local courts to observe cases being argued. For biology, they worked as volunteer docents at the local natural history museum. They not only had to absorb textbook information but also to make it understandable to younger children. The experience also provided exposure to the rudiments of public speaking.

The most popular excursion, however, capitalized on the relationship between the Recovery High program and the University of New Mexico Hospital. Robert Gougelet, the emergency medicine doctor who had become the project liaison with The Robert Wood Johnson Foundation, set up a program whereby a university hospital resident and a trained emergency medical technician came to the school to teach first aid, and linked the procedures to basic human physiology. After several weeks of classroom instruction, students took a series of week-long rotations at the hospital. They worked in the emergency room or the trauma center, in the psychiatric ward, and in pediatrics. The experiences of each rotation were fed back into both therapy and academics.

"In the neonatal intensive care unit, they'd see babies that had been born with drug addictions," Jan Hayes says. "Then they'd have to write a report on what they'd observed." The girls in particular returned wide-eyed from their tour in the unit. "Hearing them cry and seeing them born so sick and vulnerable, many of them made the connection for the first time that their drug use would gravely affect a child."

When things got busy in the emergency room, some students found themselves pressed into service, helping to set broken bones, putting pressure on wounds, assisting in suturing, and pumping stomachs. "The many patients who came in under the influence of drugs or alcohol, including some who had overdosed, had a memorable effect on the students in this rotation," Michael Hays says. "As one student put it with unintended irony, 'At first I thought this was going to be an educational experience, but then I actually learned something.'"[29]

To many skeptics in the Albuquerque school system and in the community at large, however, the goings-on at Recovery High didn't seem much like schooling, not when "young drunks" had time during the school day for recreational outings to go rock-climbing, and "teen junkies" were getting academic credit for stocking bandages in the emergency room—where they might have access to prescription drugs.

Viewed by outsiders as part leper colony, part loony bin, Recovery High occupied a peculiar place in the public eye. Community opinion was schizophrenic—people were happy to get substance abusers out of the regular public schools and away from "good, normal kids," but wanted to be sure they were not paying a premium for "coddling druggies."

—⁓— The Leaving Tree

When the target population of the school was reduced from 200 to 100 students, there was a great deal of public (and even more private) grumbling about the price tag of the program, especially about the cost per pupil and about Recovery High's staff to student ratio. Moberg and Thaler, the program's evaluators, document a total of just 208 enrollments in the program over the entire life of the school.[30] Counselor Al Sanchez's report on Recovery High puts the number of students at 366.[31] There does not appear to be any way to reconcile the two conflicting figures, and in the larger sense the disparity is unimportant. Compared with the mega-schools that typify adolescent education in Albuquerque, either figure is miniscule. With continued budgetary constraints, it's not surprising that Moberg and Thaler discovered that there was "little goodwill from many regular district school personnel toward what was perceived as an expensive program assisting few youth."[32]

The lack of goodwill contributed significantly to what Moberg and Thaler called a "failure to institutionalize." This failure was one of the major reasons that Recovery High closed. After the departure of Lou Sadler early on, no one—either within Recovery High or within the Albuquerque school system hierarchy—was specifically responsible for working toward the institutionalization and integration of the program into the district. Institutionalization didn't happen, in part because it wasn't anybody's job to make it happen.

A portion of this failure had to do with neglecting to build bridges administratively to the rest of the district—for example, not attending districtwide curriculum meetings or not interacting with other principals and counselors. There was, however, a larger financial component to the lack of institutionalization, which centered on the willingness of the school district to pay only for education and not for therapy. Since there was great effort made at Recovery High to blend the two processes, and since children entered the school with multiple substance abuse and psychological problems, it was inevitable that many believed that the school system was shouldering more than its fair share of the cost. In their post-mortem on the project, Moberg and Thaler agreed: "Given the primary treatment functions which contributed to the high costs of the program, it was unrealistic to expect Albuquerque Public School District to pick up program costs when other funding sources did not come through. From an educational perspective, the program was extremely costly and not the primary responsibility of the educational system."[33]

Nevertheless, there was some grudging acknowledgment that the Recovery High program was having an impact. Despite the multiple lapses its students had, some were returning to mainstream high schools. Of the 193 students that Moberg and Thaler were able to document, 59 returned to regular high school, and 17 returned to an alternative high school. The longer students remained at Recovery High, the better their chances for a positive outcome. Moberg and Thaler found that students deemed "successful" stayed an average of 242 days and made up 16 percent of the students who had entered the program. Those who were considered "somewhat successful" stayed an average of 157 days; these two groups represent just over half of the students who had attended Recovery High.[34]

Recovery High was always meant to be a transitional place, and one of the most moving ceremonies of the school was graduation. Students who successfully completed the program dipped their hands in paint and left their imprint on what was called "the Leaving Tree," before they departed. "One gal did her feet," Jan Hayes remembers with a grin. "Nikki was a little dynamite thing, redheaded and hot-tempered. She just hated me for the longest time. I was her nemesis, but when it came time that she finally graduated, I was the one she asked to help her put her feet up there."

At least one successful Recovery High "graduate" became a problem *because* he returned to his old school. At La Cueva High School,
Craig Fischbach had been a stellar but troubled football player, an All-
City, All-District nose tackle with a drinking problem. As fits the dual-
diagnosis profile of Recovery High students, he also suffered from
depression. After Fischbach spent what would have been his junior
year getting sober, he returned to La Cueva in 1993 as a senior, ready
to play ball. The New Mexico Activities Association (which regulates
high school sports in the state) maintained that he had used up all of
his eligibility, and barred him from the team.

Fischbach's mother, backed by the Albuquerque Public School District, brought suit, alleging that the Activities Association had violated
the Americans with Disabilities Act. The association countered that
Fischbach "is not a qualified individual with a disability"[35]—essentially contending that alcoholism was not a disease.

"The district took the viewpoint that this boy had been disabled
for a year," says Jack Bobroff, who was then Albuquerque school superintendent. "It was no different than if he'd a broken leg. When one of
these issues comes up, you always have to ask yourself, 'Is this a hill
I'm willing to die on?' The Activities Association decided they were
going to defend this hill at all costs, so they went to court."

The suit became a landmark case; the school system and the
Fischbachs won. The defeat cost the association almost $30,000 in
legal fees. Sadly, the losers blamed the Albuquerque schools in general and Recovery High in particular. "The Activities Association
spent so much money on the lawsuit that they had to increase the
dues of the members, which was every high school in the state,"
Bobroff says. "The feedback I got after that was, 'Look what you bas-
tards did! You cost us money!'"

"Costing us money" was indeed the rallying cry of those who
opposed Recovery High. There was a widespread failure, not just on
the part of the Association but on the part of the general public and
the school hierarchy as well, to understand that substance abuse is a
disease. It wasn't hard to get people to say that Recovery High was
rewarding a population of druggie losers that society had already
thrown away—and that they were doing so at the expense of a great
many more deserving youngsters.

Robert Gougelet says, "When I appeared before the school board
to ask for funds for Recovery High, I was confronted by a little old lady
in reading glasses who said, 'The school system can't afford to buy

pencils, so why should they spend $100,000 on these troublemaking kids?' It turned out she was a school librarian—and the head of the teachers' union."

Former Recovery High Board President Buzz Biernacki also recalls the acrimonious exchanges at board meetings of the public school system. "There were middle-class Anglo families saying, 'Why do I have to pay for my child's band uniform? Why can't my kid participate in wrestling? We don't have money for those programs—the school is cutting those out. How come when I look at the budget I see there's a jillion dollars for a school for some delinquent who's a substance abuser by his own choice? Tell those little punks to stop drinking and stop snorting and they won't have a problem!'"

Because Recovery High never did draw the numbers of students it had been expected to attract, the cost per pupil soared. At the time, the Albuquerque Public School District was spending roughly $2,300 per student; the cost per student at Recovery High was close to $8,000.[36] As The Robert Wood Johnson Foundation began its planned phase-out as the primary source of outside funding, the financial issue ballooned in importance.

Things came to a head in the spring of 1994, when Recovery High opponents attained a majority on the school board, and supportive superintendent Jack Bobroff retired "before they fired me." Shortly after that, Recovery High was excised from the school system's budget. In 1994, Recovery High's budget had been approximately $700,000 a year, more than half of which was provided by the public school system.

Staff and supporters of Recovery High were stunned by the sudden turnaround in their political fortunes, but mobilized quickly to fight for the school. Using the media to carry their case to the public, they tried to sway public opinion in favor of continuing the program. Parents and students picketed school board meetings bedecked in purple ribbons. (Purple is the color of recovery.) Recovering students voluntarily surrendered their anonymity and gave interviews to reporters. Alcoholics Anonymous got behind the campaign and threw its considerable resources into the effort.

Granting a reprieve of sorts, the school district finally agreed to support educational costs at Recovery High at the same rate it paid for other kids in the schools, and allocated $140,000 (the state per-pupil allotment for sixty students, or $2,333 per child) for the school. It was up to principal Jan Hayes and other supporters of the school to find the rest of the funding they needed.

In the fall of 1994, Recovery High opened for the new term, but it was a different place from what it had been before. The number of faculty and staff members was reduced, the art therapy and wilderness therapy programs were terminated, and the days and hours of operation were curtailed to be more in keeping with a conventional high school. Pressed hard by the district, the school nevertheless grew in size, but the milieu suffered accordingly.

Jan Hayes struggled to run the internal machinery of the school while she hunted for support. "I don't know how many times I went to Santa Fe, begging somebody to take this on," she says. "We would have gladly done anything to keep it open." Recovery High limped through the 1994–95 school year, but just barely. In January 1995, an emergency supplementary grant of $100,000 from The Robert Wood Johnson Foundation bailed out the program and helped keep the school in operation till the end of the school year. The Albuquerque school board chipped in $24,000 more, primarily to avoid having the school close in the middle of a semester.[37]

With funding assured through May of 1995, it looked as if the school might find enough backing to open in the fall. Supplementary state money was due to come to the school for the 1995–96 term, but in March Governor Gary Johnson slashed $36.4 million in social services programs from the New Mexico state budget, remarking that these programs "don't have a meaningful impact on our lives."[38] Among the appropriations he axed was $150,000 for Recovery High.

Recovery High closed its doors on May 25, 1995. "The Robert Wood Johnson board had visited Recovery High, and the members were very moved by the kids and absolutely knocked out by what they were trying to do there," says Foundation vice-president Paul Jellinek. "They were heartbroken when the project stopped."

They were not alone. "It was really hard to walk away," Jan Hayes says, "because we had so many kids with such new sobriety that we knew we were setting them up."

⸻ Lessons Learned

When Recovery High closed, the district instituted a program called Crossroads to take its place. Operating at two junior high schools and five district high schools, it is viewed by many as little more than a patch for ongoing drug abuse problems within the Albuquerque school system. "We've got seven Crossroads counselors, and each one of them is seeing at least a hundred kids," says Linda Orell, a substance abuse prevention and intervention specialist for the Albuquerque public school system.

"Our students were farmed out to three high schools, where they were going to have a counselor who had some background in recovery, and that person was supposed to work with the kids as they integrated back into the school," Jan Hayes says. "It wasn't very successful. After Recovery High, Al Sanchez and I worked at the Juvenile Detention Center, and we'd often see kids coming through there who'd been at the school. When they got back out, they didn't have a support system that was strong enough to keep them from going back to old behavior."

Albuquerque continues to be a center of drug trafficking; the fiscal year 2001 budget for the New Mexico High Intensity Drug Trafficking Area is $7.6 million. The Drug Enforcement Agency maintains a presence in the city, and much of its involvement focuses on an area of heavy gang activity known as the War Zone, which is roughly contiguous with the Highland High School attendance area. "This area serves the most heavily immigrant population in Albuquerque," Linda Orell says. "There are 27 languages spoken at the high school. The Crossroads counselor at Highland has a huge caseload. She can't see any student for more than twenty minutes at a time. . . . There's now an armed detective in every high school and a policeman at every middle school campus."

Rick Miera has two offices, one in Santa Fe, where he is a state legislator, the other in the Juvenile Detention Facility in Albuquerque, where he serves as coordinator of the AYUDA program. "Ayuda" is the Spanish word for "help"; it is also an acronym for Assisting Youth Using Drugs and Alcohol. "What they're doing now in the Albuquerque public schools is lip service," Miera says. "They're putting money into gang prevention—well, I'm sorry, but gang prevention is the same as drug abuse prevention. I work on this every day, and it's the same thing to me. Put a different label on it, and it's still the same problem. It's problems with kids, with families, with communication, that leads to drug abuse and gang problems. It's a mixture of all of them, and it manifests itself back where it's going to show the most— in schools—because that's where you find the most kids. That's where all this comes to roost."

Although the schools are where the problem of teenage drug and alcohol abuse is most apparent, they are not necessarily the system best equipped financially to deal with the issue—at least not without a lot of outside support. If you look just at the budget of the Albuquerque Public School District, by the numbers Recovery High was a bad deal. The school system was allotted its money from the state of New Mexico and charged with providing education for all of the children in the district. With the resources the administrators had available, they understandably felt obligated to base their decisions on the concept of "the greatest good for the greatest number." Given the $2,300 average cost per pupil for 84,000-plus children and the $8,000 cost per student of 200 to 300 Recovery High students, it's not surprising that the district was reluctant to continue underwriting the program.

"There are no villains in what happened to Recovery High," Jan Hayes says. "This is a societal problem, and it was unreasonable to expect Albuquerque public schools to do it all."

If teenage substance abuse is indeed a societal problem, then it is logical to examine the cost of treating it from a broader perspective. In 1993, the average cost per year to keep a youth interned at one of the state juvenile correctional facilities, the New Mexico Boys' School in Springer, was $30,400. The average cost per year for an inmate in the New Mexico state prison system was $28,500.[39] Few would deny that most of the students at Recovery High were headed for incarceration—indeed, many of them had already been in jail before they came to the school. From this viewpoint, Recovery High's $8,000 annual per-capita expenditure looks like a much more cost-effective investment.

"I believe that if states spent money to put schools like this together, their incarceration costs for adults would go down," says Lou Sadler, whose efforts helped to start Recovery High. "It goes for medical costs, too. Medicare and HMOs end up paying an awful lot to treat chemical dependency. If you can nip this in the bud, there would be great cost savings, but it would take several years before they'd be realized. This is the concept that I started with—'pay me now or pay me later.'"

Recovery High was one of the first schools to treat adolescent substance abuse in an educational setting, but it was not the only alternative school for recovering teens. Henderson Bay Alternative School in Gig Harbor Washington, which was visited by a delegation from Parents Against Drugs when Recovery High was in the planning stage, is still functioning. The Chicago Preparatory Charter High School in Illinois closed after just sixteen months in operation. Phoenix II High School in Gaithersburg, Maryland, is part of the Montgomery County school system, and it accommodates 30 students. The school administration has found that the average age of the student body is getting younger. Because more than 70 percent of their students are freshmen, the question of extending the program into the middle school grades is looming.

Serenity High School in San Diego was a public-private partnership institution. When the principal unilaterally fired the most popular intervention counselor in the program, drawing a storm of parent protests, it foundered in November of 1999. After it closed, the Rescu Academy, established by the fired counselor and some of the families who had been part of Serenity, opened as a private high school in nearby Santee. The newly opened academy, however, charges $10,000 per year per student. The directors hope to reduce the cost by increasing enrollment (there are now just five students) and are seeking charitable financial support.[40]

The Minneapolis-St. Paul area is home to the largest geographic cluster of alternative schools for substance abusers. Gateway School in St. Paul, Arona in Roseville, Pease Academy in Minneapolis, and Youth+Education+Sobriety (YES) in Hopkins are all small public schools. The oldest and most famous school in the area for teenagers fighting chemical dependency, however, is Sobriety High School, which was the model for Serenity High in San Diego. Opened in 1989, Sobriety High is a private nonprofit school that is under contract to the Edina School District, and claims a very high sobriety rate of 58 percent among its alumni. It receives the same per-pupil funding as other Minnesota schools, but is also supported by contributions from parents and charitable foundations. There is no charge for tuition.

The alternative schools that have survived and been successful run with small student populations—generally thirty or fewer. (Faced with a waiting list, Sobriety High, rather than increase in size, added a second, separate campus.) As was the original objective at Recovery High, all of these schools require that students be in recovery to gain admission; completion of a chemical dependency treatment program is generally a prerequisite.

In addition, these schools have generally stable populations and do not suffer the kind of enrollment fluctuations that Recovery High experienced. With the exception of Phoenix II, there is no plan made to return students to mainstream high schools. Because kids enroll and take courses with the expectation that they will graduate from these alternative schools into college or a job, disruptions to the environment due to constant comings and goings are minimized.

Most important of all, however, the successful institutions have devised means of ensuring the financial security of the school. Although these means vary from one school to another, the schools don't have to scramble on a yearly basis to remain open.

⟶ Epilogue: *Shoveling Up*

In a research program funded in part by The Robert Wood Johnson Foundation, Columbia University's National Center on Addiction and Substance Abuse, or CASA, recently completed a study entitled *Shoveling Up* that documents the cost to the public of dealing with substance abuse.[41]

CASA researchers found that nationwide, about 96 cents of every dollar spent on some aspect of substance abuse goes to dealing with the aftermath; less than 4 cents is devoted to prevention and treatment. The state of New Mexico allocates only 2 cents of every dollar on prevention and treatment. The rest of the money, almost 98 cents of every dollar, goes to dealing with the consequences of substance abuse, including juvenile justice, adult corrections, welfare, mental health, and disability. This is what the study calls "shoveling up."

"Substance abuse and addiction is the elephant in the living room of state government," says the study, "overwhelming social service systems, impeding education, causing illness, injury, death and crime, savaging our children—and slapping a heavy tax on citizens of every state." The CASA findings reinforce the concept that spreading the cost of treatment and education of adolescent substance abusers will alleviate the financial burden on local school districts, and will likely prove to be cost effective in the long term.

Notes

1. D. P. Moberg and S. Thaler, "Final Report: An Evaluation of Recovery High School," unpublished report to The Robert Wood Johnson Foundation, June 1995, p. 70.
2. High Intensity Drug Trafficking Area (HIDTA) Program, 2001 Annual Report, Office of National Drug Control Policy, http://www.whitehouse-drugpolicy.gov/enforce/hidta/nmex-main.html.

3. New Mexico Statistics, United Way of Central New Mexico, http://www.uwcnm.org/information/nmstatistics.htm.

4. *Parents Against Drugs,* "Planning Grant Proposal for Development of Recovery High School," submitted to The Robert Wood Johnson Foundation, p. 1.

5. Although Parents Against Drugs found that statistics on teen relapses were not available for New Mexico, the national recidivism rate for teens in 1990 was between 60 and 90 percent.

6. House Memorial 50 (Hawk, Hocevar), 39th Legislature, 1st Session.

7. Albuquerque School Board Resolution 89041, September 6, 1989; and Albuquerque City Council Enactment 171-1989, October 12, 1989. The language in both measures is identical.

8. M. Hays, "Recovery High School: A Program Description," Albuquerque Academy, Albuquerque, New Mexico, unpublished manuscript, p. 25.

9. D. P. Moberg and S. Thaler, "Final Report: An Evaluation of Recovery High School," unpublished report to The Robert Wood Johnson Foundation, June 1995, p. 2.

10. Ibid, p. 2.

11. Parents Against Drugs paid site visits to two other educational facilities for substance abusers. Accompanied by substance abuse professionals, they visited Henderson Bay Alternative High School in Gig Harbor, Washington, and West Valley Community School in San Jose, California.

12. D. P. Moberg and S. Thaler, "Final Report: An Evaluation of Recovery High School," unpublished report to The Robert Wood Johnson Foundation, June 1995, Executive Summary, p. i.

13. Parents Against Drugs, "Planning Grant Proposal for Development of Recovery High School," submitted to The Robert Wood Johnson Foundation, p. 7.

14. At that point, Dr. Gougelet became the project liaison between Recovery High and The Robert Wood Johnson Foundation.

15. It didn't help that after he was fired, Sadler sued the district for breach of contract, asking to be paid his $78,000 a year salary; he lost.

16. On opening day another 25 to 30 applicants were in the process of evaluation prior to admission.

17. D. P. Moberg and S. Thaler, "Final Report: An Evaluation of Recovery High School," unpublished report to The Robert Wood Johnson Foundation, June 1995, p. 42.

18. "Recovery High Implementation Summary: June 1992," unpublished report to The Robert Wood Johnson Foundation, p. 7.

19. M. Hays, "Recovery High School: A Program Description," Albuquerque Academy, Albuquerque, New Mexico, unpublished manuscript, p. 10.

20. Moberg and Thaler documented a total of 760 UAs at Recovery High, an average of 4 per student. Of these, 22% were positive. D. P. Moberg and S. Thaler, "Final Report: An Evaluation of Recovery High School," unpublished report to The Robert Wood Johnson Foundation, June 1995, p. 59.

21. The distinction was drawn by gender. Boys were official gang members; the girls functioned as a form of ladies auxiliary.

22. Recovery High School was 45% Hispanic, 33% Caucasian, 11% Native American, 2% African American, and 11% multicultural (the total exceeds 100% due to rounding). D. P. Moberg and S. Thaler, "Final Report: An Evaluation of Recovery High School," unpublished report to The Robert Wood Johnson Foundation, June 1995, p. 39.

23. A. Sanchez, "Summary Narrative Report (Descriptions/Observations): Recovery High School 1994–1995," Albuquerque Public Schools, pp. 6 and 30.

24. Ibid, pp. 6–7.

25. D. P. Moberg and S. Thaler, "Final Report: An Evaluation of Recovery High School," unpublished report to The Robert Wood Johnson Foundation, June 1995, p. 44.

26. Ibid, p. 44.

27. For budgetary reasons, the clinic was reduced in scope after the first year, and finally eliminated.

28. Center for Health Policy and Program Evaluation, University of Wisconsin-Madison, "Recovery High School Project Interim Evaluation Report," report to The Robert Wood Johnson Foundation, February 1993, Appendix A, p. 6.

29. M. Hays, "Recovery High School: A Program Description," Albuquerque Academy, Albuquerque, New Mexico, unpublished manuscript, p. 22.

30. D. P. Moberg and S. Thaler, "Final Report: An Evaluation of Recovery High School," unpublished report to The Robert Wood Johnson Foundation, June 1995, p. 36.

31. A. Sanchez, "Summary Narrative Report (Descriptions/Observations): Recovery High School 1994–1995," Albuquerque Public Schools, p. 5.

32. D. P. Moberg and S. Thaler, "Final Report: An Evaluation of Recovery High School," unpublished report to The Robert Wood Johnson Foundation, June 1995, p. 74.

33. Ibid, Executive Summary, p. vii.

34. In addition to change in alcohol or drug consumption, components of "success" for Recovery High students included improvements in knowledge

of substance abuse, social skills, self-esteem, and family communication. Ibid, p. 56.

35. "Recovering Teen Sues N.M. Group to Play Football," *Albuquerque Journal,* August 1, 1993, pp. A1 and A4.

36. Coming up with a precise per-student cost at Recovery High was difficult, because the number of students in attendance was constantly in flux.

37. "Recovery High Funded Through May," *Albuquerque Journal,* February 2, 1995, p. C2.

38 "Johnson Priorities Lock Up Our Future," *Albuquerque Journal,* March 24, 1995, p. A15.

39. New Mexico Legislative Finance Committee, Department of Education.

40. "Caring Teachers, Willing Students to the Rescue," *San Diego Union-Tribune,* May 29, 2000, p. E-1.

41. National Center on Addiction and Substance Abuse at Columbia University, *Shoveling Up: The Impact of Substance Abuse on State Budgets* (New York: National Center on Addiction and Substance Abuse, January 2001).

CHAPTER EIGHT

—∿— *On Doctoring:* The Making of an Anthology of Literature and Medicine

John Stone and Richard C. Reynolds

Editors' Introduction

In 1989, The Robert Wood Johnson Foundation funded the publication and distribution of *On Doctoring*, a book that includes short stories, poems, and essays related to medicine. Simply stated, *On Doctoring* is about setting the tone of the medical profession—a lofty goal for a simple project. While the Foundation devotes the majority of its resources to improving the organization and financing of health services, and to changing behavior and social factors that lead to poor health, grants to improve the clinical practice of medicine are still an important part of its work. Published by Simon & Schuster, the book contains writing that emphasizes the human dimensions of medical care. It is given to every student entering medical school in the United States. More than 200,000 copies have been distributed free, and thousands more have been sold to the public. The proceeds from sales are used to buy copies for future medical students. A third edition appeared in the fall of 2001.

In this chapter, the book's editors—John Stone, a cardiologist and professor of medicine and associate dean at the Emory University School of Medicine, and

Richard Reynolds, an internist, former executive vice-president of The Robert Wood Johnson Foundation, and currently courtesy professor of medicine at the University of Florida Health Science Center—offer personal reflections about *On Doctoring.* In the first part of the chapter, Reynolds reflects on how the book came to be and what it was intended to do. In the second part, Stone looks at how *On Doctoring* is put together and why chapters are selected. In the last part of the chapter, both authors reflect on the effect they believe the book has had on medical students and the practice of medicine.

Just as *On Doctoring* is an unusual project for The Robert Wood Johnson Foundation, this is an unusual chapter for *The Robert Wood Johnson Foundation Anthology.* The pieces by Stone and Reynolds illustrate how, as they wrote in their introduction to the book, "both medicine and literature have the capacity to affect the quality of the human day . . . and offer a unique view of the human condition that neither one alone can provide."

～ How the Book Began

Richard C. Reynolds

During my final year of high school, I happened to read *Arrowsmith*, by Sinclair Lewis, and *The Citadel*, by A. J. Cronin, and these two books inspired me to become a physician. My subsequent pre-med education was dominated by science courses, but also in the curriculum were two survey courses that I remember well—one in English literature and one in American literature. They introduced me to a world of writing that continues to yield discoveries. In medical school, I was the typical hard-working, compulsive student, awed by the instant intimacy of dealing with patients.

Being a doctor has always been a romance for me. It was a must for me to spend some years in the private practice of medicine, so after completing my training, I opened an office in a town of 20,000 in western Maryland. Here my education truly began. Patients came with their illnesses and in doing so told me the stories of their lives. After nine years in that practice, I spent the next two decades in academic medicine, the second as dean of the Robert Wood Johnson Medical School, a unit of the University of Medicine and Dentistry of New Jersey. In 1987, I joined The Robert Wood Johnson Foundation as executive vice-president, and remained there until 1997. Since that time I have been courtesy professor at the University of Florida. It was while I was at the Foundation that this book project began.

As it happens, there was a kind of personal literary precursor to *On Doctoring*. From 1932 to 1953, every graduating American medical student received a copy of *Aequanimitas: With Other Addresses to Medical Students, Nurses and Practitioners of Medicine* by the distinguished physician-educator Sir William Osler (who taught at the University of Pennsylvania and Johns Hopkins University, and was Regius Professor at Oxford University). Osler's book was a collection of essays about medicine—the practice, the teaching, the science, the history, and the human relationships that characterize the profession. The book was a gift from Eli Lilly and Company given to mark graduation from medical school. Pasted to the inside front cover of the book was this letter from the president of the company:

> *To commemorate the occasion we are presenting to you*
> *the accompanying volume of addresses by Sir William Osler,*
> *who followed your profession for so many years. We hope*
> *that as you read this book you will appreciate and share*
> *Sir William's inspiration, his breadth of vision, and above*
> *all, his persistent search for truth.*
>
> Sincerely,
J. K. Lilly, Jr.
President
Eli Lilly and Company

While in private practice, I was visited often by pharmaceutical representatives who promoted the products of their companies. Usually, they left brochures attesting to the effectiveness of their company's drugs. They would also give out pencils, pads, mugs, drug samples— anything to remind us of their products. I suggested to some of these representatives that their companies would be better served by providing physicians with reprints of classic medical articles, such as Peabody's "The Care of the Patient" and Beaumont's observations on gastric physiology. Some representatives were taken by this idea, but nothing came of it.

In the summer of 1987, just after I joined The Robert Wood Johnson Foundation, I wrote to 50 physician-educators across the country, asking them whether the time might be right for an anthology of literature and medicine; whether such a book would be useful to medical students; and, finally, what kinds of readings such an anthology might contain. The fundamental aim was both simple and complex: to remind medical students of the human dimensions of the distinguished profession they have chosen.

The responses were compellingly positive. There was little consensus about what readings should be included, but there was plenty of spirit behind the suggestions. Moreover, my new position at the Foundation brought me an additional opportunity: to present to its trustees the idea of an anthology for medical students. I was encouraged in this quest by Leighton Cluff, a physician who was then the president of The Robert Wood Johnson Foundation, and on December 8, 1988, I made a presentation to the Program Review Committee of the Foundation's trustees in which I described the project in the following terms:

> The current plan is to prepare a book, for the moment titled *Readings in Medicine*, which would be distributed to every student during the first year in medical school. This anthology will include essays, short stories, memoirs, and poems that describe some features of medicine of interest to a student beginning medical studies. The literature of medicine is rich in its description of individual illness and plagues, in revealing patients' reactions to illness and doctors' dilemmas in providing care. Fiction and expository forms of writing each contribute to the definition of the medical profession and the relationship of its practitioners to a larger society. Some writings portray the impressive history of medicine; others give insight into the current problems of cost and quality. Ethical controversies in research and medical practice are often brilliantly characterized in literature.

After the presentation, the chairman of the Trustee committee, Foster Whitlock, said, "Let's do it." Now an anthology had to be compiled. I would need help. Whom to ask?

Whatever success the book has had results in large part from one phone call. I had never met John Stone, but I had read some of his poems and his occasional essays that appeared in *The New York Times*. In replying to my initial letter to 50 medical educators, he had said, "Good luck on the project and do let me know if I can help further." I called and asked for his help in compiling the anthology, and he agreed.

John and I subsequently asked Lois Nixon and Delese Wear to join us in the project; they are now associate editors of *On Doctoring*. Both of these medical educators hold doctorates in areas crucial to the overall effort—literature and education—and both have long been involved in the uses of literature in medical education at their own schools. Their contributions have helped give shape and substance to the book.

In selecting work to appear in *On Doctoring*, we had, of course, a wealth of material to choose from. At editorial meetings and through correspondence, the editors discussed and debated, nominated and supported their favorite authors and literary selections. We have been unable to include some pieces of great merit because they are too long, are not close enough to the theme of doctoring, or have too much overlap with a contribution already selected. There is a conscious effort to make sure the anthology includes a diverse group of authors, with a blend of physicians and non-physicians, men and women, a mixture of poems, stories, and essays, and representative writings across historical time periods.

As we entered the final phases of the first edition of the book, we were still calling it *Readings In Medicine*, for want of a better name. We had selected the texts to be included, were making plans with the publisher, Simon & Schuster, and enjoying our work with one of that company's best editors, Frederic W. Hills. But we were still referring to the book using this clumsy name—or worse. The advertising copy that was being written used the temporary title *Untitled On Medicine*. The names we considered were just as unwieldy, and some, in retrospect, were even embarrassing.

Fred Hills was urging us to make a choice among ten or so titles "in the next few days"—time was short because jacket design was imminent. Early one morning, I had a phone call from John Stone. As he was driving to work, a possible title had occurred to him. I liked his suggestion at once and we made phone calls to all involved. There was quick and universal agreement; the title would be *On Doctoring: Stories, Poems, Essays*.

⌁ About *On Doctoring*

John Stone

The tables of contents for the three editions demonstrate that *On Doctoring* is not a static project but a dynamic one, reflecting the changing nature of the two landscapes it describes, literary and medical. For example, the third edition contains 19 new authors.

In the late 1980s, the editors came to grips with one of the first editorial problems of the first edition of *On Doctoring*: how the book was to be arranged. There was easy and quick agreement among the four of us: put the selections in chronological order by date of birth of the author. After all, life must be lived "forward," as Kierkegaard said. But we were also in agreement that we needed an opening piece to set the tone for the book, something contemporary. We found what we believed was the perfect first piece, one that appeared originally in *The New England Journal of Medicine*. Written by Dr. Carola Eisenberg, dean of student affairs (now emeritus) for many years at Harvard Medical School, the title was "It Is Still a Privilege to Be a Doctor."

In our planning for the third edition, Eisenberg's piece still seemed fresh and compelling, and remained as the opening piece. In it, she first summarizes the opposing point of view: "Indeed, some in the role of tutors for premedical students have begun to dissuade the college students they advise from choosing medicine, because they consider the prospects to be so bleak."

Eisenberg is firmly on the other side: "How absurd! It stands the world on its head to suggest that the liabilities of a career in medicine outweigh the assets. . . . The satisfaction of being able to relieve pain and restore function, the intellectual challenge of solving clinical problems, and the variety of human issues we confront in daily clinical practice will remain the essence of doctoring, whatever the changes in the organizational and economic structure of medicine." She adds, "Our students need to know about the problems facing medicine. But those problems need to be seen in perspective." She ends by saying, "What we do as doctors, most of the time, is deeply gratifying, whatever the mix of patient care, research, and teaching in our individual careers. I cannot imagine a more satisfying calling. Let us make sure our students hear that message from us."

At an editorial meeting, we decided that it would be nice to have a bookend effect in the new edition. The second edition began with Eisenberg's piece. The rest of the edition was chronologically arranged, from John Donne to Ethan Canin. What we needed to find was a companion selection to complement that written by Eisenberg—a short poem or paragraph that would be placed at the end of the book and would assert some of the same ideas her piece does. Each of us agreed, via e-mail and with some urgency, to think on this matter. That evening, while drifting off to sleep, I remembered a paragraph at the end of *As I Remember Him*, an autobiographical book by Dr. Hans Zinsser. I thought, "It just might work."

Zinsser lived from 1878 to 1940. He was born in New York City and received both his B.A. and M.D. degrees from Columbia University. He served as professor of bacteriology at Stanford, Columbia, and, finally, Harvard. His most famous work was on typhus. He isolated the bacterium that causes the disease, and, with his colleagues at Harvard, developed a way to mass-produce the vaccine. He served with the American Red Cross sanitary commission during the 1915 typhus epidemic in Serbia. His best known book is titled *Rats, Lice, and History*, a chronicling of the impact on civilization of epidemics from typhus to the black plague.

The next morning, it didn't take me long to find the selection from Zinsser's writings. As I reread the paragraph, I understood why it had stuck in my head for so many decades. Zinsser's writing was memorable both for the scene it evoked and the language he used to make his case:

> I remember one dark, rainy day when we buried a Russian doctor. A ragged band of Serbian reservists stood in the mud and played the Russian and Serbian anthems out of tune. The horses on the truck slipped as it was being loaded, and the coffin fell off. When the chanting procession finally disappeared over the hill, I was glad that the rain on my face obscured the tears that I could not hold back. I felt in my heart, then, that I never could

or would be an observer, and that, whatever Fate had in store for me, I would always wish to be in the ranks, however humbly or obscurely; and it came upon me suddenly that I was profoundly happy in my profession, in which I would never aspire to administrative power or prominence so long as I could remain close, heart and hands, to the problems of disease.

I e-mailed the selection to Dick Reynolds that evening, and he answered the next morning. "Perfect. Great find. No need to look anymore." So the third edition ends with Hans Zinsser.

All of the stories, poems, and essays in *On Doctoring* are there for a reason. The first and most important requirement is that they be well-written. Beyond that, we have chosen some selections because they have proven useful in the classroom or because they can trigger specific discussions, often ethical in nature. The short play "Fortitude," by Kurt Vonnegut, was included in the second edition and remains in the third. It is a provocative piece, with the biting dark humor one expects of this author. The machinations of its characters asks the reader to consider the ever-changing world of biotechnology as it seeks to provide "life support" for failing organs.

The selection, "Misery" by Anton Chekhov, illustrates the power of *On Doctoring* to direct the attention of medical students beyond the scientific to the personal and emotional. The story begins with an epigraph: "*To whom shall I tell my grief?*"

Only a few pages long, "Misery" concerns one Iona Potapov, driver of a horse-drawn carriage on a blustery and snowy night. As Iona ferries three different groups of passengers, he tries to tell each of them about a great loss he has suffered: his son has died this week, in a hospital, victim of a fever. The passengers, though, are oblivious, some drunkenly oblivious, to Iona's plight. Listen to Chekhov's description:

"*But the crowds flit by heedless of him and his misery. His misery is immense, beyond all bounds . . . His son will soon have been dead a week, and he has not really talked to anybody yet . . . He wants to talk of it properly, with deliberation . . . He wants to tell how his son was taken ill, how he suffered, what he said before he died, how he died. . . ."*

Distraught, Iona ends work early and leads his little mare to the stable, saying, *"'Since we have not earned enough for oats, we will eat hay.'*

Iona is silent for a while, and then he goes on:

'That's how it is, old girl. . . . Kuzma Ionitch is gone. . . . He said goodbye to me. . . . He went and died for no reason. . . . Now, suppose you had a little colt, and you were mother to that little colt. . . . And all at once that same little colt went and died. . . . You'd be sorry, wouldn't you? . . .'
The little mare munches, listens, and breathes on her master's hands. Iona is carried away and tells her all about it."

For the most part, we have preferred that selections in *On Doctoring* be complete in themselves. When this is not possible, we have chosen compelling chapters from longer works. One good example is the excerpt from Dr. Abraham Verghese's book *My Own Country*. The book chronicles the effects of AIDS on a town in Tennessee, where Verghese served as a specialist in infectious diseases. The excerpt points up the human dramas that surround AIDS and leads to discussions of its attendant problems: complex ethical issues; the cost of sophisticated health care; the disruptions of family units; the ways in which society cares for (or doesn't care for) the terminally ill.

The writers gathered in *On Doctoring* deal with the medical profession, of course, but their other, inseparable theme is that of humanity. Anatole Broyard, the late editor and essayist, who wrote a *New York Times Magazine* piece called "Doctor, Talk To Me" about his own illness, prostate cancer, and his difficulties in finding a physician to treat it, puts the matter this way:

Not every patient can be saved, but his illness may be eased by the way the doctor responds to him—and in responding to him, the doctor may save himself. But first he must become a student again; he has to dissect the cadaver of his professional persona; he must see that his silence and neutrality are *unnatural*. It may be necessary to give up some of his authority in exchange for his humanity, but as the old family doctors knew, this is not a bad bargain. In learning to talk to his patients, the doctor may talk himself back into loving his work. He has little to lose and much to gain by letting the sick man into his heart. If he does, they can share, as few others can, the wonder, terror, and exaltation of being on the edge of being, between the natural and the supernatural.

Because poems are short and evocative and can communicate a complete experience in a few words, they recommend themselves for the anthology. Poems can be squirreled away in the crevices of time between a medical student's readings in biochemistry and physiology. Listen as the American poet, James Dickey, describes a patient's encounter with diabetes:

Diabetes

I

Sugar

One night I thirsted like a prince
Then like a king
Then like an empire   like a world
On fire. I rose and flowed away and fell
Once more to sleep. In an hour I was back
In the kingdom   staggering, my belly going round with self-
Made night-water, wondering what
The hell. Months of having a tongue
Of flame convinced me: I had better not go
On this way. The doctor was young

And nice. . . .

"Diabetes," from *The Eye-Beaters, Blood, Victory, Madness, Buckhead* by James Dickey, copyright © 1968, 1969, 1970, by James Dickey. Used by permission of Doubleday, a division of Random House, Inc.

And who has given better counsel to surgeons than Emily Dickinson?

> Surgeons must be very careful
>
> When they take the knife!
>
> Underneath their fine incisions
>
> Stirs the Culprit—*Life*!

In the third edition of *On Doctoring*, after considerable debate, we selected authors, agreed on a new cover, and included a new section called "Suggestions for Further Reading." The suggestions were made by teachers of literature and medicine at medical schools across the country. The list is not exhaustive, but is meant to convey something of the wide variety of readings that commend themselves to a medical student throughout a career in medicine.

Some of our suggestions may seem startling at first glance—Mary Shelley's *Frankenstein*, for instance, or Kafka's *The Metamorphosis*—but they have all been found provocative and compelling in unique ways. Tolstoy's *The Death of Ivan Ilych* is as admirable and important a rendering of the stages of dying as those summarized by Elisabeth Kubler-Ross. Albert Camus' *The Plague* begins with an attack of bubonic plague in a city in Algiers; before it concludes, it has raised profound questions about all plagues. Other suggested readings on the list include *Death in Venice*, by Thomas Mann; *The Doctor's Dilemma*, the play by George Bernard Shaw; *Awakenings*, by Oliver Sacks; *Tuesdays with Morrie*, by Mitch Albom; and *Middlemarch*, by George Eliot. And, of course, *The Citadel* and *Arrowsmith* are on the list.

Our youngest contributer is Gregory Edwards, who, at the time I first read his poetry, was ten years old, a fourth grade student at Robert Shaw Traditional Theme School in the DeKalb County Schools in Georgia.

The Department of Medicine at Emory University had "adopted" the school. One evening in December, 1999, several faculty members gathered at the mostly-minority school to meet some of the teachers and hear students perform a series of skits. After the skits, we adults began to visit our assigned rooms. I was directed to Ms. Dunn's room, whose fourth graders were well prepared for this event. Her class had been studying poetry and for the evening's event, some of her students had written poems. Ms. Dunn had put together a booklet of her children's poems, and had bound them with ribbon in a bright yellow plastic cover signed by all the kids and emblazoned, "Happy Holidays, Dr. J. Stone." I was impressed, and decided to read several short poems in the booklet for the class gathered around me. I gave each poem in turn my best declamatory effort.

When I came to the poem by Gregory Edwards, I asked Gregory to raise his hand. He was a handsome young man with a broad smile. I liked his poem very much and relished reading it aloud.

The Shot

Going to the doctor
With my father.

The scary, scary doctor!

Dad's gonna get a shot.
He's as stiff as a robot!

The scary, scary doctor!

We are getting closer.
We are in.

The scary, scary doctor!

He got his shot.
All that was left was a dot.

Several days later, at work on the next edition of *On Doctoring*, I was reminded of Gregory Edwards' poem. I decided to send it around to the other editors, with the recommendation that we consider it for inclusion in the next edition. Why? Because the poem captured so well a child's perceptions of going to the doctor, especially that most-dreaded part of the encounter: "the shot." Because of its sense of drama and its sense of humor. Because it portrayed the intimidation that all of us, young and old, experience when we see our doctors. Because it captured the magic patients hope for from their doctor, that magic bullet delivered without pain. And because, after all is done—and said—it was a good poem.

The editorial judgment was unanimous. Gregory's poem should be included. I called his school and told his teacher, Carole Dunn, who told Gregory, who told his mom. Not long afterward, Dunn called to say the principal had invited me to the next PTA meeting so the whole school could celebrate Gregory's triumph.

The auditorium was packed. Gregory and I sat in little plastic chairs in the front row. Suddenly, I was being introduced. I gave a brief history of the book project to the audience, and mentioned some of the familiar names in the table of contents. "So, next edition, Gregory's name and Gregory's poem will be in this book, along with some other pretty famous writers such as Robert Frost and Alice Walker." The audience rose in unison and applauded.

I told the audience something of my own reaction to Gregory's poem—how it used rhyme, meter, suspense, and humor, all to great advantage. I asked Gregory if he thought his poem was funny. He nodded "Yes" and told the audience why: "I think it's funny because it was my father who was going to get the shot, not me!"

⌇⌇ The Impact of *On Doctoring*

Richard C. Reynolds and John Stone

Foundations want to know whether their contributions make a difference. But how does one measure the impact of giving *On Doctoring* to each new medical student? Do such students become better doctors? Can this be measured? We know of no satisfactory way to answer these questions. We can note, with pleasure, that over the past decade we have received many letters from medical students attesting to their appreciation of the book. For some, it has been invaluable as a diversion from their ponderous textbooks. Others report a better understanding of the social aspects of medical practice, and still others a keener insight into how patients struggle with their misery and how doctors attempt to provide relief. We recently received a letter of thanks signed by all members of the freshman class at one medical school. The mother of another student wrote of the satisfaction she gained by reading her son's copy of *On Doctoring*. It gave her a better awareness of the challenges medicine would offer her son. Personal testimony alone, however, no matter how generous, cannot always be equated with worthiness.

To recognize entry into the medical profession, many medical schools have developed a "White Coat" ceremony for new medical students. Early in their first year, the students attend a convocation in which they don their white coats, sometimes are presented with a stethoscope, and may participate in the taking of oaths (such as the Hippocratic Oath) about being a physician. This assembly is used by many schools as a setting in which to distribute *On Doctoring*. In recent years, there has been a national upsurge in the teaching of humanities at medical schools. Assigned reading from *On Doctoring* has become a mainstay in these courses. The inclusion of the book in medical education confirms our biased perception that the book is worthwhile. And the book still strikes us as the right thing to do. That may be all the justification that is needed.

A Look Back

CHAPTER NINE

—⁓— The Foundation and AIDS: Behind the Curve but Leading the Way

Ethan Bronner

Editors' Introduction

The emergence of AIDS in the early 1980s challenged many of the tenets of grant-making that characterized the Foundation's approach of that period, particularly its reluctance to focus on specific diseases. By the mid-1980s, the dimensions of the AIDS crisis, the lack of leadership from government and the philanthropic community, the potential impact of the disease on the nation's hospitals, and the urging of leading public health experts across the country led the Foundation to rethink its position. In 1986, the Foundation announced the first of its programs aimed at mobilizing resources and public opinion to combat AIDS.

The initial program followed a preferred Foundation approach to grantmaking: find a model of service delivery that looked promising—in this case it was the San Francisco model—and then test it at a number of other locations in the hope that the federal government would adopt and expand it. The Foundation subsequently funded an open-ended nationwide program seeking innovative ways of preventing HIV/AIDS (especially in low-income communities, where most AIDS patients contracted the disease through substance abuse), a public television series, and many individual projects.

Despite its initial reluctance to enter the field, The Robert Wood Johnson Foundation became the largest source of philanthropic funds devoted to AIDS prevention during the late 1980s, and became known for its work on AIDS. The Foundation's first president, David Rogers, was named vice-chairman of the National Commission on AIDS in 1989 after leaving the Foundation.

In this chapter, Ethan Bronner, the education editor of *The New York Times*, chronicles the way in which the Foundation responded to the AIDS crisis. It is a story of how one foundation dealt with an area of high sensitivity and, in the author's words, "how AIDS changed The Robert Wood Johnson Foundation [and] also, in an important sense, how AIDS changed the country."

The patient is a 30-year-old black man with daunting medical and social problems. He is thin, and suffers from nausea, chronic fatigue, and pain in his feet and hands. He walks with difficulty. He is on a cocktail of medications that he obtains from several different providers, telling each a different story. He is seeing a psychiatrist but misses appointments. His t-cell count is low, his viral load high. He lives with his parents but they are throwing him out. He has AIDS.

On an oppressively hot Tuesday afternoon in August, 2000, Carla Gray, a case coordinator at AIDS Arms, in Dallas, enters a large meeting room at the Cathedral of Hope in the city's Oak Lawn section. She needs the kind of coordinated help for this patient that cannot be had through a phone call or two. It is at this weekly meeting—and only at this meeting—that such help is available to Dallas's AIDS patients. Seated there are representatives from several dozen community service groups, among them the AIDS Resource Center, HOPWA (Housing Opportunity for Persons with AIDS), and Parkland Hospital's Amelia Court Clinic, which has the largest number of AIDS cases of any area hospital. Gray presents the case, starting with the medical and moving to the social. Then she lays out what must be done. Her patient needs food and housing. His medicines (both psychiatric and for HIV) need to be straightened out and to come from a single source. He could also use clothing and transportation. Before the hour is out, she finds him a room to share, secures a commitment from a food pantry, and settles on a clinic and a social worker. He will be picked up for his psychiatric sessions. Later the same day, she will speak to her patient's physician and psychiatrist.

Such AIDS case management meetings have taken place every Tuesday afternoon in Dallas since 1986, when, with a grant from The Robert Wood Johnson Foundation, the Community Council of Greater Dallas set the program in motion. At first, of course, the meeting was much smaller. Fewer groups were represented, and fewer cases were discussed. It was held not in a large room at the Cathedral of Hope but in a small one at St. Thomas Episcopal church. Two other differences are especially noteworthy. The cases then under consideration contained virtually no African-Americans or women. The cases were those of gay white men. And perhaps most significant of all, the goal was different. Today, AIDS case management involves medical treatment using protease inhibitors and retroviral agents that help patients to live. Then the aim was the much grimmer one of helping patients to die.

In the year 2000, some 5.3 million people around the world, including 600,000 children under the age of 15, became infected with the HIV virus that causes AIDS, according to the World Health Organization. It has killed about 22 million people, including 3 million in 2000. And the number of women dying from it exceeded the number of men in 2000. The epidemic has been especially fierce in sub-Saharan Africa, home to 10 percent of the world's population and 72 percent of new AIDS infections.[1]

In the United States, AIDS has gone from a disease of largely gay men to one affecting the poor and intravenous drug users. And it has turned from an unambiguous death sentence to a chronic condition that can be managed. About 1 million people in the United States and Canada are living with the virus, with approximately 45,000 new cases of AIDS in the year 2000.

Despite those changes, the kind of community-based case management launched in 1986 with Foundation grants totaling $17.2 million in Dallas and 10 other communities around the country has held up remarkably well, and continues without significant structural or conceptual shift. Although more and different kinds of organizations are involved, the typical patient has changed, the Foundation has moved on, and the programs are paid for today with federal and state funds, the community-based case management approach remains an integral part of scores of urban and rural health networks.

"The Robert Wood Johnson Foundation played a key role," remarked Philip Lee, a former assistant secretary of health in Democratic administrations who was instrumental in getting the Foundation involved from his position at the University of California at San Francisco. "Here we saw this thing going on with what appeared to be very serious implications, and we were appalled that the government and foundations were doing nothing."

What The Robert Wood Johnson Foundation did was this: noting that San Francisco, through community-based groups, had found a way to care for AIDS patients more effectively and humanely outside hospitals, it paid to create similar four-year demonstration projects in 11 communities through a project called the AIDS Health Services Program. The sites were Atlanta, Dallas, Fort Lauderdale, Jersey City, Miami, Nassau County, Newark, New Orleans, New York City, Seattle, and West Palm Beach. The idea was to get others (either foundations or the state and federal governments) to match the grants and take over the programs. That, by and large, happened. Shortly after the first Foundation grants were made, they were matched by federal emergency funds set aside for AIDS, and in 1990 Congress passed the Ryan White Comprehensive AIDS Resources Emergency Act, which authorized funds for programs based on the Robert Wood Johnson model.

In 1988, the Foundation's involvement in AIDS took two more turns. As the nation was gripped by the spreading epidemic, with tens of thousands dead and dying, the Foundation invited proposals from anyone for anything related to AIDS care. The response was overwhelming. More than 1,000 proposals came in from organizations in 48 states, the District of Columbia, and two territories, with requests ranging from $1,000 to $10 million. Almost the entire staff of the Foundation spent weeks sifting through the proposals. More than 80 percent of the requests came from communities outside the major epicenters of HIV infection—Los Angeles, New York, and San Francisco. Leighton Cluff, then the Foundation's president, issued a statement at the time to Congress and the public saying, "We knew that few community-based AIDS projects qualified for existing federal, state, or private funding, particularly those located in low-prevalence areas. Now we've documented the extent of that funding gap and the nature of the problems these communities are confronting." Dozens of groups were funded, including those engaged in educating runaway youths in the Southeast, union members, and a network of interfaith volunteers coordinated by Associated Catholic Charities of New Orleans.

In the same year, some $4 million went to a four-part PBS series called "AIDS Quarterly," hosted by Peter Jennings. The idea was to reach millions of viewers with a reliable broadcast focusing on scientific, public policy, legislative, and community elements of AIDS. The series was produced by WGBH in Boston, which is responsible for the NOVA and Frontline programs.

With all these projects funded—and several others, including a pediatric AIDS program at Yeshiva University in New York—the involvement of The Robert Wood Johnson Foundation in AIDS had become enormous. Indeed, a paper published in August, 1990, by senior Foundation staff members declared, "The Robert Wood Johnson Foundation has awarded over 100 AIDS-related grants totaling more than $45 million, making it the single largest source of private philanthropic funding for AIDS to date."[2]

One year later, the Foundation largely withdrew from the business of funding new AIDS projects, both because it worried that it was getting involved too deeply with a single disease and because federal funding for AIDS had finally taken off, allowing for a graceful exit.

While it may seem self-evident today that what was then the nation's largest health care philanthropy would take on the nation's largest epidemic, this was far from a certainty at the time. After the disease was first identified, four years went by without the involvement of Robert Wood Johnson or, for that matter, any other national foundation. And once The Robert Wood Johnson Foundation did decide to play a role, many were surprised. As Frank Karel, a Foundation vice-president, put it, "I was frankly astounded—pleased but astounded—when we went into AIDS. It represented a sharp departure and carried so much baggage." The story of how the Foundation made the decision to enter the AIDS maelstrom, and was changed by it, is a complex one. It is partly the story of how the Foundation grasped what was still an unarticulated precept: that to make a difference in health, it would often have to consider social issues far from medicine per se. It would also have to be willing to take a risk. How AIDS changed The Robert Wood Johnson Foundation is also, in an important sense, how AIDS changed the country.

—⁓— The Epidemic Emerges

Epidemics often begin surreptitiously. On June 5th, 1981, the *Morbidity and Mortality Weekly Report* of the Centers for Disease Control, gave the first published notice of a new syndrome by describing five homosexuals afflicted with pneumonia at three different California hospitals. "The fact that these patients were all homosexuals suggests an association between some aspect of a homosexual lifestyle or disease acquired through sexual contact and pneumocystis pneumonia in this population," the report noted. Over the next few years, that pneumonia and Kaposi's Sarcoma, a previously rare skin cancer, became achingly familiar manifestations in thousands of gay men of what was named Acquired Immune Deficiency Syndrome.

Homosexuality may not yet be fully accepted in American society, but it is such a widely recognized phenomenon today that prime-time television shows, whole areas of study, and even some college scholarships revolve around it. Vermont now legally sanctions civil union between two men or two women. Few can be unaware today that there is an active gay community in the United States; it is an increasingly mainstream viewpoint that homosexuals should have the same rights as heterosexuals. Yet when AIDS broke out, homosexuality was still a sufficiently taboo topic that the disease was largely ignored. It made everyone uncomfortable. As Randy Shilts wrote in *And the Band Played On*, his classic account of the early AIDS years, "From 1980, when the first isolated gay men began falling ill from strange and exotic ailments, nearly five years passed before all these institutions—medicine, public health, the federal and private scientific research establishments, the mass media, and the gay community's leadership—mobilized the way they should in a time of threat. The story of those first five years of AIDS in America is a drama of national failure played out against a backdrop of needless death."[3]

There were three reasons not to expect The Robert Wood Johnson Foundation to jump into AIDS care. First, the Foundation, which began its work as a national philanthropy in 1972, had decided from the outset not to focus on any single disease. It viewed single diseases as the province of the National Institutes of Health and of disease-specific voluntary agencies like the American Cancer Society and the American Heart Association.

Second, having chosen to focus on health service delivery, the Foundation saw no obvious role for itself in an epidemic that seemed primarily to require biomedical and clinical research, epidemiological surveillance, and public education.

And finally, for a conservative board of directors that was still entirely male and white, there was the specter of controversy. It can be hard to remember today, in a country that has heard public discussions of oral sex in the Oval Office, but throughout the first part of the 1980s, with President Ronald Reagan in office, public dialogue was not open to issues of sexuality, let alone homosexuality. Edward N. Brandt, Jr., assistant secretary for health in the Department of Health and Human Services in the first Reagan administration, recalled talk among fellow federal officials that AIDS was "God's vengeance" for immoral behavior.

"The room would have cleared if someone said they had AIDS," he added. "On television, I couldn't use certain phrases to describe how the virus is transmitted, because that might offend the American public, and we had whole meetings about how to refer to sexual intercourse."[4]

Many complained at the time that Reagan and his aides rarely spoke publicly about AIDS, thereby adding to the public's tendency to ignore the spreading epidemic. But Brandt says he takes partial responsibility for the silence and, in retrospect, believes that it was the right path. "My sense was that if Reagan and those around him had spoken about AIDS, it would not have been helpful. I figured the best thing to do was to depoliticize it by telling them we should leave it to the doctors and scientists."

As late as 1985, the CDC had stopped spending money on AIDS education because the White House had worried that the government ought not to be funding what, in its view, amounted to instructions in male anal intercourse. According to Shilts, the CDC director, James Mason, was heard to complain that he had suddenly found himself talking with complete strangers "about sexual acts that he would not discuss with his wife even in the privacy of his own home."[5]

Steven Schroeder, president of The Robert Wood Johnson Foundation, said it was no surprise to him that the board had not jumped in earlier. "When I came on as president, in July of 1990, I was the youngest of 18 white men on the board," he said, noting that today four members are female and black or Hispanic. "Foundations tend to be conservative and not to take risks. And the population with AIDS was a population that the Foundation's board was not very familiar with."

Robert Blendon, a professor of health policy at Harvard University, who was the Foundation's senior vice-president in the mid-80s added, "We went through 10 years convincing people we were not a single disease foundation. We used to have to explain this to board members who had concerns of their own like prostate cancer or heart disease. So how do we explain that this one is different? Older Americans were the last ones to worry about AIDS. This was not a disease that affected them or their friends. And they were less likely to be open to other ways of life. So although the Foundation's staff wanted to get involved, it seemed impossible at first."

By the summer of 1985, however, the epidemic had forced its way into the national consciousness. More than 20,000 Americans were either dead or dying of AIDS. And one of those, it turned out, was Rock Hudson, the square-jawed leading man in scores of films like "Pillow Talk" and "Magnificent Obsession." The news that the actor who played the quintessentially American romantic man had "the homosexual disease" produced a groundswell of attention. President Reagan, a former actor, suddenly connected to this disease. He called Hudson in his Paris hotel room to wish him well (Hudson, ashamed of his condition, had gone to Paris for treatment) and Ed Brandt, who had been a Reagan administration official, said colleagues told him this was a big turning point in the federal government. Hudson became the hook for numerous media organizations to focus on AIDS in a serious way for the first time. The disease was front-page news in virtually every major newspaper on Sunday, July 28th. That week, both *Time* and *Newsweek* produced large stories on Rock Hudson and AIDS.[6]

All of the public discussion of AIDS increased the sense among Foundation staff members that they could no longer sit this one out. Other pressures to act had been building as well. Ruby Hearn, a senior Foundation vice-president, recalls a talk to Foundation staff members in 1984 by the Princeton sociologist Paul Starr after the publication of his book, *The Social Transformation of American Medicine.* Starr said that the public response to AIDS was shamefully lax, and urged the Foundation to do something about it.

Starr noted that the response of others elsewhere to his view on AIDS was indicative of the era. "In a speech to a group of health care executives, I spoke with some passion about the need for a concerted response to the AIDS epidemic," he recalled. "Someone from the audience asked me, 'Are you married?' I was. The questioner assumed that anyone who cared about AIDS was gay. One of the huge barriers to an effective response was precisely that many people didn't think AIDS was a matter of 'public health.' They thought it involved the health of a 'special interest,' and of course they blamed the epidemic on moral conduct they disapproved of."

But beyond the growing urgency and public attention, something significant took place that gave the Foundation the opening its staff sought. A new study showed that the way the San Francisco gay community had organized itself to cope with AIDS was making a big difference for the city's overtaxed hospitals and for the patients themselves.

⁓ The AIDS Health Services Program

As early as 1982, a multidisciplinary outpatient AIDS clinic was set up at San Francisco General Hospital, and by 1985, the concept of community-based services for people with AIDS had emerged in the form of a locally organized collaborative network of hospitals, outpatient clinics, and volunteer-driven community-based groups. Care was coordinated by case management, which included emotional support, counseling and advocacy in obtaining home care, hospices, and public health education. According to studies carried out then and later, those factors were primarily responsible for dramatically reducing the average length of a hospital stay for AIDS patients. That stay was 11.7 days in San Francisco compared with 25.4 days in New York City, where outpatient community-based care did not exist.

Such coordination of care was not entirely new or unique. It had been used successfully in San Francisco and elsewhere for the mentally ill after the de-institutionalization wave of the 1970s, and for the elderly. But urban hospitals, already overtaxed by the crack epidemic and still-rising crime, were faced with an acute burden as AIDS patients started to fill their wards. AIDS patients often lost their jobs and their insurance and became dependent on Medicaid. The hospitals were threatened with becoming their homes. Here Foundation staff members saw a way to bridge their concerns about AIDS with the traditional ones of their board.

Drew Altman, president of the Henry J. Kaiser Family Foundation in California, was at the time a vice-president of The Robert Wood Johnson Foundation and recalls being goaded by his wife to find a way for the Foundation to get involved.

"I discovered that in San Francisco they had developed a model that could be applied to the rest of the country," he recalled. "The way the Foundation worked was to find a model, replicate it, and evaluate it. David Rogers was president of The Robert Wood Johnson Foundation at the time, and he was nervous about this because of the single disease question. But when he saw how the San Francisco model could be used to help save teaching hospitals, he saw a way to sell this to the board. He understood that we could say, 'Hey, Hopkins and others could go down the tubes. So we need to help the teaching hospitals, not just gay people.'"

Patricia Franks, director of the AIDS Resource Program at the University of California, San Francisco under Philip Lee, remembers Lee, accompanied by Mervyn Silverman, director of public health for San Francisco, approaching David Rogers. They told him that the government was doing nothing, there was no funding for this epidemic, and Robert Wood Johnson could play a key role. They were armed with a study they had commissioned showing that AIDS patient care in San Francisco was significantly less expensive than elsewhere because of its community-based approach.

The key meeting to bring the Foundation into AIDS care occurred in the fall of 1985, when Lee and Silverman came to the Foundation's Princeton headquarters. Silverman and Lee made their case well. They had data, and they had a plan that could be replicated. And those items were what Rogers and his staff needed. It was not hard to make the case decisively at the next board meeting, where the plan was approved. As John Gagnon, a sociologist and an expert in the fields of sexuality and AIDS put it, "The Robert Wood Johnson Foundation was as slow to respond as everyone else but it was on the cutting edge of that slow response."

In the following year, cities with heavy AIDS caseloads worked to put together proposals based on the San Francisco model. In late 1986 and early 1987, the successful proposals were selected, and the grants were distributed. From the start, it was clear that San Francisco offered a model, but only in the most general sense. Other cities had AIDS, but they did not have the highly organized and professional gay community of San Francisco. In fact, by the time the Foundation's work began, the disease had already peaked and started to subside in San Francisco. Sexual practices that spread the disease, including indiscriminate partnering at bathhouses, had declined markedly. And politically San Francisco was extremely well organized. So to use it as a model was fine as a start, but far from perfect.

In the two-city project of Newark and Jersey City in New Jersey, for example, AIDS was never a gay epidemic but—foreshadowing a nationwide pattern that would emerge 5 to 10 years later—a disease of intravenous drug users and their sexual partners, including many non-whites. Steven Young is today deputy director of the Office of Science and Epidemiology at the HIV/AIDS bureau of the Health Resources and Services Administration, or HRSA, in the U.S. Department of Health and Human Services. In 1986, as a state employee, he served as project director for the Foundation-funded project for the two New Jersey cities. Young said recently, "When I came to the federal government in 1990 and people were starting to talk about the changing demographics of the epidemic, I said, 'What are these people talking about?' The AIDS patients in the city where I come from were 75 percent intravenous drug users."

New Jersey set up case management meetings in a dozen different medical care settings to discuss coordination and efficiency, as Dallas had done. Newark was already facing an AIDS epidemic among children, he recalled. But the biggest challenge was organizing the various elements of the community.

"It was not an easy sell," Young said. "We primarily addressed issues from the perspective of medical care—establishing clinics to deal with the throngs knocking on the doors of the ERs—and working through substance abuse centers. We had a very difficult time getting the more traditional black community-based groups and churches to really recognize the issue."

Not having that community base was not exclusively a bad thing. It meant less public support, of course, but it also allowed for greater direction from the top. "When people are not as well organized, there is less political opposition to each step," Young said. "You could simply create things because they were needed and then bring people along."

Young sees the Foundation-supported work in New Jersey as largely successful but not entirely so. "I don't think we ever proved that we were able to reduce hospital use in New Jersey," he said. "The idea was that by setting up an individual care plan, patients wouldn't use the hospital as much. In fact, we found the cost overall going up because we gained access to services for people who had been outside the system. Not surprisingly, if you include more people, it costs more."

Cost aside, community-based case management can be a tricky business, as other communities discovered. Robert Blendon, the Harvard University health policy researcher and former Robert Wood Johnson Foundation senior vice president, said that the organization of care was challenging. "In a hospital you are lying in your bed and hundreds of things are given to you," he said. When patients are in a community setting instead of a hospital, he explained, there are a series of independent organizations providing care, and a central group to coordinate services is needed. "And don't forget that in many of these cases we were talking about a population that feels discriminated against, so you had to include them in the decision making. There was a constant feeling on their part of being experimented on, the way African-Americans in the South used to feel," Blendon said.

Yet how to include intravenous drug users? This was not a notably well-organized community, nor was it easy to serve them. As Merv Silverman put it, "It is easier to put gay men in housing than someone who is shooting up."

Relations between and within groups were delicate. Warren W. Buckingham, known to all as Buck, works today on AIDS as a senior technical adviser in the Africa bureau of the United States Agency for International Development. He began his long career in AIDS when he started the Dallas AIDS ARMS program ("ARMS" is an acronym for "Accessing Resources to Mobilize Support") in 1986.

"In the gay community in Dallas, there had been almost no cooperation between men and women," Buckingham said. "A lot of gay men were sexist. Eventually, they got over that, because lesbians with nothing to gain saw their brothers dying and stepped up and provided the care."

In some projects, there were uneasy relations between the administrators and sectors of the affected population. Many recall, for example, that in a major Southern city, a society woman ran the AIDS outreach program. She worked well with gay men but not with poor African-Americans. And in Dade County, Florida, the heavily affected Haitian community vigorously opposed listing Haitians as "high-risk."

Many of the community-based organizations that got involved in AIDS case management were born specifically for that purpose, often starting with nothing more than a telephone in someone's living room. They sometimes failed to mature into real organizations, making care somewhat sketchy. As John Gagnon, the sociologist who studies AIDS, described the situation, "There were lots of fake community organizations, a kind of pseudo-grass-rootsism." But he acknowledged that it was not clear what the alternatives might have been.

Indeed, evaluating the effectiveness of a program aimed at a crisis is difficult, because when one asks if something worked, the reply must begin with "Compared with what?" Vincent Mor of Brown University's Department of Community Health was commissioned by the Foundation to lead a team of evaluators after the AIDS Health Services Program was under way. They reported, "High caseloads limited case managers to providing what amounted to information and referral services to many clients, and prevented case managers from monitoring their clients as frequently as desired. Case managers were forced into a mode of responding to crises and 'putting out fires': Opportunities for proactive—rather than reactive—intervention were thereby restricted. In this respect, the AIDS Health Services Program did not provide a strong test of case management for people with AIDS because in many locations the intervention was not implemented in an optimal manner."[7]

In conclusion, the Mor team pointed to the tensions between minority and non-minority community groups, the attention that needed to be paid to keeping tense consortia together instead of treating patients, and the gap between plans and reality.

"The broad goals of all the AIDS Health Services Program consortia as articulated in 1986 were lofty, ambitious, and unattainable—and reminiscent of earlier efforts at social reform," the evaluators said.[8] They added that it might make sense, over the long term, for consortia responsibility to be assumed by a lead agency, but that the agency should not become a new bureaucracy.

But Mor and his colleagues did note that the Ryan White Comprehensive AIDS Resources Emergency Act of 1990, named for an Indiana boy who struggled heroically with AIDS, was modeled directly on the Foundation-sponsored projects. The Ryan White Act drew on the project's approach in a number of ways. This included the use of a case-management, community-based model of care intended to relieve hospitals, the use of representative community planning groups and development of local political leadership, the use of volunteer/ buddy support and community-based organizations for a variety of health and supportive services, and the focus on maximizing the availability of all local, state, and federal funds to develop a comprehensive continuum of care.

Yet another important contribution of the AIDS Health Services Program was in personnel. Many of the key players in federal AIDS care—Pat Franks, Buck Buckingham, Steven Young, Andy Kruzich of Seattle—gained vital experience in the field with the Foundation's projects.

The Robert Wood Johnson Foundation, in keeping with its policy of creating a demonstration project and then getting out so that others may take it over, built its exit into AIDS Health Services after four years. It funded only those projects which could demonstrate that they had found other sources of support for the following years, and Foundation officers also urged the federal government to supplement and extend its funds. In 1986, partly in response to the Foundation's efforts, Congress appropriated and the Health Resources and Services Administration, or HRSA, funded four cities—Los Angeles, Miami, New York, and San Francisco—for a total of $15.3 million. Over the next few years, the federal government added more, some of them also served by the Foundation. By 1989, HRSA funding covered 25 communities, including all the Foundation-funded sites.

Many of the projects around the country were chagrined when the Foundation kept its word and declined to renew them. Pat Franks at the University of California at San Francisco was one of them. She recalls in 1988 trying hard, in conjunction with Philip Lee, to persuade the Foundation to renew its grant. When that failed, the two of them wrote a long letter of thanks detailing how the money had been useful.

"I was disappointed, but they did a good thing because the government needed to see that this couldn't be done by a foundation,"

Franks said. "They also felt that if they continued to put huge amounts of money in, nobody else would get into the game. The Ford Foundation got involved in a limited way and so did local and regional foundations. But the real point was to get the federal government involved, and that is what happened."

⟿ The AIDS Prevention and Services Program

Part way through the AIDS Health Services Program, Foundation staff members saw a growing need for additional AIDS-related activities. As time went by, it became clear that there were multiple causes of AIDS and that it was not unique to the gay community. In March, 1988, the Foundation issued an unprecedented Call for Proposals. Unlike any of its previous Calls for Proposals, this one set no overall funding level and had no time or dollar limit for individual grants. Foundation vice-president Ruby Hearn recalled, "For the first time in our history, we put out word that said, 'Give us your good ideas on how to deal with this.' We were inundated with requests."

The Foundation gave applicants just under four months, until July 1, to apply. As Leighton Cluff, then the Foundation's president, put it in a special memorandum to congressmen and state officials, the Call for Proposals had two purposes: to generate imaginative ideas for the Foundation to consider, and to provide a measure of the nation's unmet demand for help in fighting the epidemic.

The response was 1,026 proposals totaling more than $537 million over periods ranging from three months to six years. Especially noteworthy was the fact that many proposals came from places not traditionally associated with AIDS—like Fargo, North Dakota, and Cheyenne, Wyoming. Proposals came from churches, schools, and the Girl Scouts. Nearly a third of the proposals targeted minority groups. One of the applications was written in Spanish; others proposed producing bilingual and culturally sensitive materials. And just under half of the applications sought funds for efforts to prevent the further spread of HIV infection.

The Foundation awarded $16.7 million to 54 projects together called the AIDS Prevention and Services Program. The projects included an AIDS prevention program for primary and secondary school students in Anchorage, Alaska, that used native puppets and familiar role models in Alaska Native culture; a prevention program for migrant farm workers in Delaware, Maryland, and Virginia; an education and outreach program for homeless people in Los Angeles;

and a service, referral, and day care program for infected mothers and their children in Boston.

Project Street Beat, sponsored by Planned Parenthood of New York City, sent mobile medical vans to reach out to teenage prostitutes, young intravenous drug users, and homeless young people in the South Bronx and Brooklyn. Its director, Jeanne Kalinoski, said, "We know they aren't going to come in and ask for help, so we go out to them." Another project provided AIDS education to working prostitutes in Denver and San Francisco. Still another offered dental care for HIV-infected people and another free bedside legal information. Yet another offered information and referrals to AIDS patients who had lost their sight, a fairly common but unnoted problem.

One of the enormous shifts in American society produced by AIDS was that, because of the necessity to educate the public on the spread of the disease, discussions of sexual practices had become nearly commonplace. Merv Silverman, the director of public health in San Francisco at the start of the AIDS epidemic, remembers designing the first anti-AIDS poster in 1982. It was viewed as scandalous at the time. It simply urged gay men to reduce the number of their partners and not to take drugs. Six years later, in a sign of the changed times, as part of the AIDS Prevention and Services Program the Foundation was sponsoring projects in which teenagers lectured one another on the use of condoms by spreading them over fruits and vegetables.

Some of the projects were good and successful; others were less so. There developed a sense in the Foundation that this kind of approach—funding that is broad but thin—has limited impact. But the experience of trying to plug holes in the care and education provided to those with AIDS gave the Foundation's staff members a sense of how to move forward as a philanthropy. They noted that irrespective of the kind of physical or mental disorder suffered, the impediments encountered were pretty much the same—uncommunicative bureaucracies, uncoordinated services, insurance benefits that were poorly designed for people with chronic conditions, and case managers being funded only rarely, even though they are often the glue in the system.

By the 1990s, the Foundation had changed its grantmaking approach with respect to chronic conditions and was tackling systemic problems in the way services were organized and provided to people with chronic disorders.

ᗧ AIDS Quarterly

One other significant project of the late 1980s was "AIDS Quarterly," the PBS series hosted by Peter Jennings. The project's four broadcasts were widely described as among the most powerful and frank discussions of the epidemic on American television. When Jennings introduced the first installment, in the winter of 1989, he laid out the grim statistics: "45,000 people are dead so far and 1.5 million of our fellow citizens have the AIDS virus." He added, "Every minute, someone on our planet gets the AIDS virus."

One of the broadcast's main tasks was to dispel prejudices and myths, to make clear that AIDS is a disease, not a providential plague, and to fill a hole left by the delinquent media. "Let's get one thing clear at the outset," Jennings said. "AIDS is a virus. It is not a moral issue. And another thing. We in the media have not always been very helpful to you in understanding AIDS." He then laid out some of the frequent misconceptions about the disease that had been repeated on major news broadcasts—for example, that AIDS can be transmitted by mosquitoes or kissing.

"AIDS Quarterly" offered a mixture of longer documentary pieces and shorter, snappier moments of scientific and political update, like the controversy over whether to make the experimental drug AZT more available despite the concerns of the Food and Drug Administration. Among the more powerful segments was one that followed Admiral James Watkins, chairman of a committee appointed by President Reagan to make recommendations on AIDS. Called "The Education of Admiral Watkins," the segment showed a churchgoing, strait-laced admiral who had never before met an AIDS patient or thought much about the disease traveling to AIDS clinics and parts of the inner cities like New York's Hell's Kitchen.

"We had our own biases unrelated to reality," the admiral acknowledges of his committee and himself partway into the documentary. The segment showed the admiral learning that hemophiliac children who had contracted AIDS through blood transfusions faced fear and prejudice in their own communities because of the unfounded belief that other children could be infected simply by playing with them. In Anderson County, Tennessee, for example, a 12-year-old boy was banned from school. "This was in the Bible Belt," Admiral Watkins says in sad wonderment. "Where are our pastors? Where are our religious leaders?"

Another segment showed the Pacer family of Salt Lake City, a large Mormon family of seven grown children and 35 grandchildren. Joe Pacer, the family's head, was a doctor and a highly respected community member. His fourth child, Malcolm, 39 years old, was gay and had contracted AIDS. The segment showed the family obliged to reconcile its own feelings toward homosexuality, forbidden in the Mormon church, and its love for Malcolm, who died at the segment's conclusion. As Jennings said after that segment, the broadcast's aims were, in part, to "dispel myths and allay irrational fears."

While many agreed that the broadcasts were first-rate, others raised the question of how effective they were on a network that tends to draw largely educated viewers. Others countered that informing and winning over the élite is a vital task in any campaign. No one sought to measure the program's impact. Given the difficulty of measuring the effectiveness of educational broadcasts such as the "AIDS Quarterly," its impact remains unclear.

—— Looking Back: The Foundation's Role in the AIDS Crisis

The Foundation largely ended its direct support for AIDS care with the end of the AIDS Health Services Program in 1991. By then, federal programs ran into the billions, and there was no longer a clear need for a trail-blazing effort on the Foundation's part.

"I didn't feel any push from anyone to go forward with AIDS funding," Steven Schroeder says of his arrival as the new president in July of 1990. "No one came up with a version 2.0 of it. There was lots of federal funding for it by that time, and the role of a foundation like ours is not to pile on."

The Robert Wood Johnson Foundation still plays an indirect role in AIDS through its programs on drug abuse and the homeless. Its Faith in Action program supports local coalitions of congregations providing volunteer aid to those who are homebound. About 10 percent of those are HIV-positive, according to Schroeder.

Paul Jellinek, the Foundation vice-president who helped to begin the Foundation's first AIDS project, recalls well the difficulties caused by religious objections to homosexuality. Lessons from those early days are applied today in many programs, including Faith in Action. Among other things, Jellinek said, there is special value in getting churches to help those with AIDS: "It helps debunk the 'wrath of God' argument. If churches are stepping up to the plate, it sends a different message. That's one of the things you learn with experience."

There were other lessons as well. Foundation officials understood at the outset that San Francisco's AIDS health care model could not be replicated precisely because of the unique circumstances of that city and its well-organized gay community. But using it as a model still offered lessons about the difficulty of taking an approach to one kind of community and bringing it to entirely different circumstances. Community-based care models were far more complicated in Newark and Jersey City, because where there were so few gay AIDS patients and so many intravenous drug abusers, a very different kind of "community" existed. It also turned out that creating community-based organizations in loose-knit communities was more easily said than done.

The AIDS Health Services Program brought the Foundation into an area where it could make a difference. For a variety of reasons, the federal government was staying out; other foundations were nervous about getting in. The Robert Wood Johnson Foundation saw an opportunity and seized it. It offered a model for helping patients and relieving hospitals that the federal government adopted, setting the stage for the Ryan White Act. At the same time, the Foundation saw the opportune moment to leave the scene and devote its energies to other areas. Finally, in examining the AIDS Health Prevention and Services Program, officials of the Foundation saw the limits of making grants to many groups dealing with different elements of the disease. It refocused its efforts afterward to try to have more systemic impact, an approach that has been the dominant one in recent years.

Notes

1. "AIDS Infections Rise Globally, but Sub-Saharan Cases Stabilize," *New York Times*, November 25, 2000, p. A5.
2. P. S. Jellinek, R. P. Hearn, and L. E. Cluff, "Responding to AIDS: The Robert Wood Johnson Foundation's Experience" in *AIDS and Public Policy Journal*, *August*, 1990, p. 212.
3. R. Shilts, *And the Band Played On* (New York: St. Martin's Press, 1987), p. xxii.

4. "Proceedings of AIDS Prevention and Services Workshop," unpublished report of The Robert Wood Johnson Foundation, February 15–16, 1990, p. 36.

5. R. Shilts, *And the Band Played On* (New York: St. Martin's Press, 1987), p. 586.

6. Ibid, p. 578.

7. V. Mor, J. A. Fleishman, S. M. Allen, and J. D. Piette, *Networking AIDS Services* (Ann Arbor, Michigan: Health Administration Press, 1994), pp. 89–90.

8. Ibid p. 208.

Inside the Foundation

CHAPTER TEN

~ Program-Related Investments

Marco Navarro and Peter Goodwin

Editor's Introduction

This chapter is one in a series that looks inside The Robert Wood Johnson Foundation. Past volumes of the *Anthology* have examined the Foundation's research and communications strategies, its core values, and the thinking that led it to address substance abuse. Here, Marco Navarro, a program officer at the Foundation, and Peter Goodwin, the Foundation's treasurer, discuss a little-known philanthropic tool: program-related investments, or PRIs.

A PRI is essentially a loan. The loan approach can be appropriate when an organization realistically expects its initiative to generate enough income to repay the loan—for example, by buying a building that will bring in rental income. Most often associated with the Ford Foundation and the MacArthur Foundation, which pioneered their use, PRIs have become more common as the assets of foundations have increased. From 1998 to 1999, PRI authorizations nationally jumped from $203 million to $267 million—a rise of 31 percent. Still, PRIs represent only a small percentage of foundations' awards; in 1999, the nation's 50,000 foundations distributed $23 billion in the form of grants.[1]

In the world of foundations, the current buzz term is "venture philanthropy," which means that foundations adopt a businesslike attitude and explore how their investments can bring about measurable payoffs in terms of social outcomes. PRIs are, in a sense, precursors to this venture philanthropy approach.

Why would a foundation such as Robert Wood Johnson, with more than $8 billion in assets, make a loan as opposed to an outright grant to a struggling nonprofit trying to develop an initiative? In this chapter, Navarro and Goodwin address this issue as they examine The Robert Wood Johnson Foundation's experience with PRIs.

1. L. Renz, "PRI Financing: 1998–1999 Trends and Statistics," in J. Falkenstein, editor, *The PRI Directory* (New York: Foundation Center, 2001).

Foundations are a uniquely American phenomenon.

They allow the private wealth of individuals and organizations to be transferred to institutions working to promote the public good. By federal law, foundations must pay out at least 5 percent of their assets every year for charitable purposes. Virtually all of this "payout" is in the form of grants, but there is another, less well-known mechanism that foundations can use to carry out their charitable purposes: loans, or, as they are more formally called, program-related investments.

— Program-Related Investments: The Historical Context

In the Tax Reform Act of 1969, Congress created the concept of program-related investments, or PRIs. As defined in that law, a program-related investment is an investment (usually a loan) that meets three requirements:

- Its primary purpose must be to accomplish charitable objectives.

- It cannot have, as a significant purpose, the production of income or the appreciation of property (i.e., a prudent investor seeking a market return would not enter into the investment).

- It cannot be used for lobbying or to support lobbying.[1]

As long as a PRI meets these requirements, it can be counted, as grants are, toward meeting the 5 percent payout required by law. PRIs enable foundations to (1) stretch their resources (since they can recover the principal and sometimes receive interest); (2) fund projects, such as building construction, that are not usually considered appropriate for grant funding; and (3) invest in high-risk charitable ventures or borrowers that commercial banks tend to avoid.

Although a PRI may generate interest income, it is conceptually very different from a foundation's regular investment portfolio. The objective of a PRI is to further a foundation's charitable purposes, while the objective of a foundation's investment portfolio is to preserve capital and to produce market-oriented returns.

Over the past 30 years, a number of foundations have utilized PRIs, although mainly on a limited basis. Among foundations that regularly make PRIs, the Ford Foundation has invested 2 percent of its assets, the John D. and Catherine T. MacArthur Foundation 1.5 percent, and the Irvine Foundation 1 percent.[2]

~~~ When Loans Make Sense

Four different circumstances can trigger the consideration of PRIs as a funding mechanism.

First, activities that will produce income for the borrower that can be used to repay the loan are prime candidates. Most commonly, PRIs are used to finance the construction or rehabilitation of buildings that can be rented. Since The Robert Wood Johnson Foundation generally will not provide grant funds for bricks and mortar, PRIs offer a way to finance building construction. They have also been used to provide student loans that can be repaid upon graduation and to support medical practices in underserved areas that can be repaid out of revenues from patient-care.

Second, the lack of credit-worthiness of many nonprofit organizations makes them suitable candidates for PRIs. Banks are often unwilling to make loans for real estate transactions to nonprofit organizations because of their slim operating margins, uncertain funding, inexperience with loans (or finances generally), and lack of resources that can be used as collateral. Foundations can step in and make loans to nonprofit organizations that commercial lenders consider too risky.

A third circumstance in which a PRI can make sense is as a source of gap financing. A dollar gap can appear at any stage of a project. For example, at an early stage, foundations can provide the seed money needed to shape an idea, explore its feasibility, and begin pre-development work such as hiring an architect—elements that often must be in place before banks will consider financing a project. Or, once a project is under way, a PRI can be used to provide bridge financing that will take it from one stage to another.

Fourth, where a program calls for loans to a number of community organizations, it might be appropriate to make a PRI to an intermediary organization that in turn will make smaller loans to fund a number of projects. In this way, a foundation can stretch its limited dollars, spare itself the administrative burden of supporting and evaluating a multitude of small borrowers, and tap into existing development and financial expertise.

⟶ The Robert Wood Johnson Foundation's Experience with PRIs

The Foundation's first PRI, made in 1982, was a $3 million loan to the United Student Aid Funds, to be used as collateral for scholarships for needy women and rural and minority medical students. Its most recent PRI was made in 1997—a $1 million loan to help the Minneapolis Foundation establish a program expanding medical services in underserved rural and urban areas.

The Foundation has made 26 loans, totalling $35 million. Of this, $16 million was awarded to organizations participating in national programs that included both a grant and a loan component. The remaining $19 million was in loans for programs that had no grant component. A significant amount of the loan portfolio went to establish statewide or national loan programs that then provided credit to many smaller nonprofit organizations. Over the years, the Foundation's experience with PRIs has been more the product of seizing specific opportunities than of forward planning.

PRIs to Finance Building Construction and Renovation

Most PRIs have been made to enable the recipient to put together financing needed to construct or renovate buildings, such as community mental health facilities, hospitals, skilled nursing and long-term care facilities, and day-care housing.

THE COMMUNITY HEALTH FACILITIES FUND

The Community Health Facilities Fund, or CHFF, is a not-for-profit organization that enables community-based behavioral health care organizations to gain access to tax-exempt debt financing by pooling their loan applications. The idea grew out of a national survey conducted in the late 1980s that found an unmet need of nearly $2 billion for the capital costs required to build and renovate treatment facilities for people with mental illness, substance abuse problems, and developmental disabilities. Most organizations providing services were nonprofits whose limited experience, low cash reserves, and tenuous revenue streams hindered their ability to obtain capital financing. It seemed logical that if the organizations' loans could be grouped and the risk spread among them, then investors would be more likely to buy the bonds the group would issue.

Building on this suggestion, in 1991 the Foundation awarded a $5.5 million PRI to establish the Community Health Facilities Fund. The loan was to be paid back with 2 percent interest over a 25-year period. A second loan for $2.8 million was made in 1995.

The loan program went through two phases. The first, between 1991 and 1995, blended traditional bond financing and the concept of group risk-sharing. In Illinois and Florida, bonds were issued to pay for capital improvements and a 10 percent reserve was set aside to cover bad debt. Government agencies reviewed the applications to assure program eligibility and the financial strength of the applicants. The problem was that some of the organizations applying for loan funds—for example, a small clinic needing to expand—were not financially strong enough to attract investors. The solution was to put both strong and weak applicants into a single pool before making the bond offering. The Robert Wood Johnson Foundation's PRI to the Community Health Facilities Fund was used to add an additional 10 percent to the reserve fund to cover defaults, thus making a total of 20 percent set aside to cover bad debts. This additional 10 percent (known as "credit enhancement") gave investors the security of knowing that their risk of losing money was further reduced. Florida raised $23 million and Illinois $7 million in municipal bond offerings.

The second phase, from 1995 to the present, dealt with two problems that were recognized early by CHFF and Foundation staff members. First, organizations needing loans were not usually ready for pooling at the same time, yet the concept required that they all had to be presented to potential investors simultaneously. Second, the approach taken in the first phase was limited to the states in which the offering was made. This precluded national offerings or placing organizations from different states in the same pool. In response, CHFF created a trust instrument that grouped loan applications from a number of organizations throughout the country as they became ready and placed them into a single loan pool. Within the pool, loans were then divided according to risk. The less risky loans were packaged and sold to traditional investors. The riskier loans were held and backed by the Foundation PRI.

To date, the PRIs, totaling approdimately $8 million, have enabled CHFF to help 30 community-based behavioral health organizations throughout the United States secure approximately $85 million in loans to construct new buildings, renovate facilities, and buy equipment. The tax-exempt debt, which nonprofit organizations are able to obtain through the CHFF, provides them with lower interest rates, more capital, and longer repayment periods than commercial lenders are able to offer. It is one of the few programs to give nonprofits access to this kind of flexible, low-cost, and long-term credit. Moreover, according to Chris Conley, the president of Connecticut-based Nonprofit Capital LLC and manager of the CHFF, "PRIs have created a model for delivering a certain type of capital to the nonprofit behavioral care market. The tax-exempt bond market is not set up to finance large numbers of unrated nonprofit corporations that have relatively small capital needs. The CHFF program has created a structure and process to do that."

CHFF loans are paid back through the patient revenue streams. To date, there has not been a single default. The program has demonstrated that nonprofit organizations, even those without a significant credit history, do repay their loans.

THE PROGRAM ON CHRONIC MENTAL ILLNESS

In 1986, the Foundation launched a national Program on Chronic Mental Illness. It funded the creation of Local Mental Health Authorities in nine locations to coordinate the care of people with serious mental illness. The needs of this population include health care, support services, and housing so that they can remain in the community. The Program on Chronic Mental Illness was funded largely with grants, but there was also a PRI component. Loans of $1 million, payable over 10 years at 4 percent interest, were made available to each of the program's sites.

All nine sites took advantage of PRIs. Since the Local Mental Health Authorities were concerned mainly with providing clinical services, and did not, as a rule, have expertise in housing or mortgage financing, Local Housing Development Organizations, linked with the Local Mental Health Authorities, were set up to acquire and rehabilitate housing, to place clients, and to manage the properties. The loans were made to these Local Housing Development Organizations. They, in turn, entered into partnerships with state mental health or financing agencies and used the loans to buy and renovate properties. Most were small family units; even residential complexes were small, with the largest being 4 to 6 units. After the properties had been acquired, the states provided grants and long-term mortgage financing. State funds helped to retire the loans so that additional properties could be acquired. The participation of the U.S. Department of Housing and

Urban Development in the program lowered the risk of default. It agreed to provide 125 rental subsidies through so-called "section 8 certificates" for each of the nine sites.

Through the PRI mechanism, the Program for Chronic Mental Illness was able to leverage $9 from federal, state, and private sources for every dollar lent by The Robert Wood Johnson Foundation. To date, over 4,500 units have been developed. The former national deputy director of the program, Martin Cohen, observed that the PRIs made it possible "to sustain large amounts of affordable and safe housing for people with serious mental illness. Already, other organizations and groups (and others without experience) that serve an array of disabled and disadvantaged people who lack needed housing and supports are using this model." All loans due have been repaid.

AIDS HOUSING OF WASHINGTON'S BAILEY-BOUSHAY HOUSE
In 1990, the Foundation awarded AIDS Housing of Washington a $1.5 million PRI, payable over 10 years at 3 percent interest, to help finance its Bailey-Boushay House. Located in Seattle, Bailey-Boushay House was the nation's first newly constructed skilled-nursing and day-health facility for people with HIV and AIDS.

When the 3 percent interest rate of the PRI was combined with the higher market rate of a commercial bank loan, the overall long-term borrowing rate decreased to a manageable 8 percent. This saved Bailey-Boushay House about $500,000 in interest payments over its first ten years of operation, and helped assure the long-term viability of the facility. Bailey-Boushay House has served more than 2,000 people with HIV/AIDS in its 35-bed facility and day health program. The loan has been fully repaid.

OUR COMMUNITY HOSPITAL
A PRI to Our Community Hospital, in Scotland Neck, North Carolina, provided the financing needed to transform itself into a long-term care facility and offer the kind of services needed by its aging population.

Our Community Hospital, in rural northeast North Carolina, was in danger of being closed because the number of patients had decreased and the amount of red ink had increased. In 1989, the citizens of the Scotland Neck decided to convert the hospital to an extended care facility, complete with senior housing, swing beds (which could be used for short- or long-term care), and a primary care facility.

Lacking experience in this kind of transaction, the community turned to the North Carolina Office of Rural Health for assistance. The Office of Rural Health sent an advance team to determine the feasibility of a conversion and to identify sources of financing. The feasibility study yielded a "go" decision. Revenues were expected to come primarily from federal and state governments once the facility was designated as a rural health clinic under federal law.

In 1990, The Robert Wood Johnson Foundation made a $500,000 PRI to Our Community Hospital. The loan was used to fill various gaps in financing the conversion. The state of North Carolina provided matching funds, and the community conducted an old-time fundraising campaign, complete with sales of books, candles, and cookies. Our Community Hospital continues to thrive and to meet the health care needs of its community. The loan from The Robert Wood Johnson Foundation was repaid in 2001.

PRIs to Finance Medical and Nursing Practice in Underserved Areas

Loans have been used to finance physicians and other health professionals who agree to set up practices in underserved rural or inner-city areas. Two PRIs are particularly noteworthy: Practice Sights, a national program that encourages health professionals to work in underserved areas, and the hospital-based rural program of West Alabama Health Services.

PRACTICE SIGHTS: STATE PRIMARY CARE DEVELOPMENT STRATEGIES

In the 1990s, the Foundation began to address some of the structural and social factors that discourage health care professionals from practicing in rural areas and inner cities: poor reimbursement, isolation, and the lack of social amenities and professional opportunities for health professionals and their spouses. In 1992, the Foundation initiated Practice Sights: State Primary Care Development Strategies, a five-year program to increase the number of primary care providers in medically underserved areas. Under this program, ten states were awarded grants to train physicians, nurses, and other providers, and to give them incentives (such as forgiving loans and providing assistance in practice management) to work in rural areas and inner cities. In addition, a loan component was added and earmarked largely for the construction, renovation, and equipping of facilities.

Every Practice Sights grantee was eligible to apply for a PRI. After a competitive application process, the Foundation made 10-year, 3 percent interest loans ranging from $700,000 to $1.5 million to applicants in four states. Each of the loan recipients was required to raise five dollars from other sources for every dollar of PRI funds it received. Two states, Virginia and Idaho, designated nonprofit agencies to receive and manage PRIs. They, in turn, placed the loan proceeds in bank certificates of deposit. The banks committed themselves to make loans under their most flexible terms and to manage this portfolio of loans themselves. The two other states, Nebraska and Minnesota, designated nonprofit agencies to receive and manage the PRIs directly. In Nebraska, an area economic development agency agreed to match the Foundation loan on a 5-to-1 basis and to underwrite and manage the loan portfolio. In Minnesota, a community foundation agreed to a similar matching, underwriting, and loan management agreement.

According to an assessment conducted by the Practice Sights National Program Office, the PRIs produced mixed results.[3] The Healthy Communities Loan Fund of the Virginia Health Care Foundation, which received the first and smallest loan of $700,000, in 1995, has made 16 loans totalling nearly $1.6 million. These have helped recruit 24 primary care providers (physicians, dentists, nurse practitioners, and physician assistants) to areas needing health professionals. In November, 2000, the project's banking partner, First Virginia Bank, received the Main Street Award from the American Bankers Association's Center for Community Development for its work in this project. Minnesota, which received a $1 million PRI in 1997, has made $1.1 million in loans to date, largely for capital improvement projects.

The two other states—Nebraska and Idaho—have since closed their loan programs and repaid the loans. Both states indicated that the loans were too stringently structured: They felt that the 5-to-1 matching requirement was too high, that the 3 percent interest rate charged by the Foundation was not competitive, and that the loans should have been made for more than 10 years.

WEST ALABAMA HEALTH SERVICES, INC.
In 1991, The Robert Wood Johnson Foundation made a $500,000 PRI to West Alabama Health Services, located in one of the more medically underserved areas in the country. Attracting health profession-

als to the region is a great challenge. The West Alabama Health Services, a nonprofit organization dedicated to providing health care for people in the region, took an innovative approach to the workforce problem. It decided to borrow money and capitalize a leasing company. Unlike, say, an automobile leasing company, which rents a product, the West Alabama Health Services leasing company employed people—doctors, nurses, respiratory therapists, midwives, and other professionals—whom it rented to underserved communities. The idea was that the leasing company would be able to guarantee a salary to its health professionals, thus attracting them to West Central Alabama. In turn, the community clinic would use patient revenues to make lease payments to the West Alabama Health Services leasing company. Lease payments would then be used to repay the Foundation loan.

The concept was unique to the area, and no other funders or lenders would participate. However, the project had two crucial factors working for it. First, the organization and its director, James Coleman, have a long history of delivering on projects. Second, the organization had an unusual form of collateral. In the event that West Alabama Health Services could not meet payment on its note, it pledged revenues from the Greene County Racing Commission, which oversees the dog tracks that are extremely popular and lucrative in Alabama.

PRIs to Guarantee Student Loans

In earlier days, the Foundation used PRIs to guarantee loans that enabled deserving women and minority students to attend medical school to become health professionals. The United Student Aid Funds, a recipient of grants from The Robert Wood Johnson Foundation since the mid-1970s, made loans to needy African-American, Native American, Hispanic, and women medical students. By 1982, there were enough defaults on these loans that the United Student Aid Funds was worried that its reserve fund might be depleted. It requested a grant from the Foundation to increase the reserves. However, the Foundation did not feel that grant funds were appropriate, and agreed to provide the United Student Aid Funds a $3 million interest-free PRI to be used as a reserve against default on the student loans. The PRI was repaid and closed.

Hybrid Grant-Loan Arrangements

Although mechanisms that combine elements of grants and loans are not specifically loans, they do bear a sufficient resemblance to PRIs to merit discussion. These hybrid options are relatively new to the Foundation's work. "Recoverable grants"—non-interest-bearing funding instruments—are one of these mechanisms. The Primary Care Development Corporation received a recoverable grant. Similarly, the Foundation has made grants to organizations that have, in turn, used the money to establish revolving loan funds. The NCB Development Corporation does this to provide pre-development and bridge financing to organizations constructing affordable assisted living facilities, and the Southern Rural Access Program does it for the purpose of increasing access to primary care in rural areas of the South.

THE PRIMARY CARE DEVELOPMENT CORPORATION

In 1993, the Foundation awarded the New York City–based Primary Care Development Corporation, or PCDC, a $1.5 million grant and, in 1996, a $300,000 recoverable grant as part of an ambitious multifoundation effort to establish a new agency whose goals included developing 40 new or expanded primary care centers and increasing the ability of health care providers and staff to effectively run these centers. A total of $35 million from a variety of public and philanthropic sources supported PCDC's operations, $17 million of which came as a grant from New York City to establish a pre-development revolving loan fund. PCDC would eventually have access to more than $250 million in municipal bond financing for the primary care centers; in addition, PCDC provides a wide range of technical support services to the staffs of the centers.

The recoverable grant helped PCDC pay personnel and other costs while it waited to receive financing and fees it had charged its clients for its services. The fees were to reimburse PCDC for the staff time and other expenses associated with helping clients obtain loans. Under the terms of the recoverable grant, PCDC would begin repayment of the principal 16 months after its award. It would pay the Foundation 10 percent of its positive cash flow starting in June, 1998, and the monthly payments would continue until the principal was fully repaid.

By the end of 1999, PCDC had helped to expand or build 28 health centers, representing a total investment of $100 million. However, the nature of the financing it carried out had changed considerably. Most notably, there was an increased demand for smaller loans. Loan requests from smaller, less experienced organizations require much more assistance in helping clients understand and prepare financing applications. Also, smaller agencies, with less of a track record, have less chance of getting financing than larger, more established applicants. Thus, more PCDC staff was needed to spend more time providing technical assistance to agencies that had less chance of actually getting funded. Since fees are paid only on projects that are approved, the revenues received fell well short of projections. In 1999, the Foundation agreed to forgive the recoverable grant and thereby waive the repayment of the funds.

NCB DEVELOPMENT CORPORATION

In 1992, the Foundation authorized a national program called Coming Home, and it gave the NCB Development Corporation, the national program office, a $6.5 million grant to develop model affordable assisted-living facilities for low-income and frail seniors in rural areas. The NCB Development Corporation used $4.3 million, or about 70 percent of its grant, to establish a revolving loan fund. This fund had originally been conceived as a source of permanent financing capital that organizations would then leverage with other forms of permanent financing.

As the Coming Home program developed, however, it became clear that the loan funds would be better spent in a project's early stages on market research, planning, and other predevelopment work. Banks generally are reluctant to provide loans for these purposes, especially to nonprofits with little real estate experience. Yet they are critical. David Nolan, the director of the Coming Home program, noted, "These costs can easily reach $125,000 and very few not-for-profit community-based organizations have that kind of money to risk. But without spending that money, no project would ever happen. It was the classic Catch-22 situation, but one that the revolving loan fund could remedy."[4] So the plan shifted and the revolving loan fund was used to enable nonprofits to borrow money in order to pay for feasibility studies, marketing surveys, other pre-construction costs, and bridge financing to prevent delays between different stages of a project. According to Nolan, the revolving loan fund has helped produce 330 affordable assisted-living units and leveraged nearly $32 million in equity, secondary financing, grants, and conventional debt for eight projects.

SOUTHERN RURAL ACCESS PROGRAM

In 1997, the Foundation funded the Southern Rural Access Program to help build the institutional and leadership capacity necessary to improve access to basic health care in eight of the nation's most medically underserved rural states. In part, the program provides grant funds that can be used to establish revolving loan funds designed to help rural doctors, other providers, clinics, and hospitals gain better access to capital financing sources.

Virtually all the projects started in early 1999, so information about the program is limited. However, two states, South Carolina and Arkansas, have already approved more than $4 million in loans, and the projects have been able to secure matching support from a variety of sources, including the U.S. Department of Agriculture (Arkansas, Louisiana, South Carolina, and West Virginia); state government (Louisiana and West Virginia); private philanthropy (West Virginia), and community development financial institutions (Arkansas and Mississippi). All the projects intend to work closely with the private banking community, and to leverage additional capital resources from it.

An interesting feature of the Arkansas and Mississippi projects is the selection of not-for-profit intermediaries—the Arkansas Enterprise Group and the Enterprise Corporation of the Delta—that know economic development and capital financing in distressed rural communities and are now adding health care lending. These organizations' knowledge of capital financing, and their strong working relationship with federal financing sources—including the Department of Agriculture, the Small Business Administration, the Department of Treasury's Community Development Financial Institution program, and the New Markets Tax Credit Initiative, which was just passed by Congress—could create some interesting models in the next several years.

—— Conclusion

Twenty years and $35 million later, what can be said about program-related investments as a way of carrying out The Robert Wood Johnson Foundation's mission—or, for that matter, any foundation's mission? What lessons have been learned, and what changes should be considered?

> First, PRIs are an appropriate, and underused, mechanism for foundations.

Loans allow a foundation to finance nonprofit organizations that want to build or renovate real property or to attract health professionals to underserved areas. Although traditional lenders are often not interested in taking a chance on such high-risk borrowers, this is exactly the kind of risk-taking for the public good that philanthropic organizations were designed for.[5]

In addition to making capital available for projects that are otherwise unattractive to commercial lenders, PRIs have been shown to enhance the financial skills of the nonprofit organizations that borrow money. Negotiating and managing PRIs have provided them the experience on which to build subsequent projects. PRIs that enable small nonprofit organizations to buy a building also give them a sense of security, since they no longer have to worry about rent increases or finding new space if a lease runs out.

Second, the Foundation's experience has demonstrated that nonprofit organizations, even struggling ones, do repay loans on time.

The repayment record of the nonprofits has been excellent. As commercial lenders see that nonprofits pay back their loans on time, they are likely to be more willing to support projects at earlier stages of development.

Third, PRIs are difficult for both foundations and the organizations seeking loans.

For a foundation, PRIs are time-consuming, require a great deal of paperwork, and have legal and financial implications (such as due diligence requirements) that grants do not require. Foundations are not generally set up to operate as banks, but PRIs put them in the position of acting as bankers. PRIs also raise ethical issues: for example, can a foundation, in good conscience, foreclose on a failed loan to a nonprofit organization doing good work?

For an applicant, gaining access to foundation loans can be difficult. Negotiating a loan agreement requires time and skills that many nonprofits may not possess. On top of that, on any single project an applicant may have to juggle financing from several sources, each with different terms and conditions.

Fourth, the terms, such as interest rates and length of a loan, are sometimes onerous; flexibility should be built in.

In a number of cases, interest rates fell nationally afer PRIs had been made, and loans could be obtained on more favorable terms than the Foundation had been able to offer. However, borrowers were locked in to the terms that had been negotiated earlier—and had since become non-competitive. In addition, a 10-year repayment period might have been too short, given the length of time it takes to develop the loan programs and the high cost of maintaining them. Making loans that bear no interest and have longer repayment periods—20 to 25 years, say—would alleviate these problems. In addition, consideration should be given to reducing stringent matching requirements, without compromising the Foundation's interest in leveraging other funds.

Fifth, PRIs should include some grant funding for marketing, technical assistance to borrowers, and loan administration activities.

Generally, the cost of aggressively marketing the loan program, hiring a staff to help organizations apply for loans, and servicing the loans was not taken into account when the repayment terms were negotiated. These are legitimate expenses that benefit borrowers and insure that the PRIs are maximized and used as intended.

In its two decades of experience with PRIs, The Robert Wood Johnson Foundation has tried a variety of approaches. They range from the relatively simple, such as gap financing for Our Community Hospital in rural North Carolina, to the more complex, such as pooling applicants for tax-exempt bond issues in the Community Health Facilities Fund and supporting a company that leases health professionals in rural Alabama. Even now, the Foundation is trying new hybrid approaches that combine grants with loan financing. There does not appear to be a single model that works best, and perhaps that is an advantage. PRIs can, and should, be flexible enough to meet the needs of borrowers and the marketplace.

Notes

1. Internal Revenue Code section 4944(c) as summarized by J. Weiser and F. Brody, *Introduction to Program-Related Investments*, http://www.brodyweiser.com/articles/IntroPRI.html.

2. J. Weiser and F. Brody, *Introduction to Program-Related Investments*, http://www.brodyweiser.com/articles/IntroPRI.html.

3. North Carolina Foundation for Advanced Health Programs, *Assessment of Practice Sights: State Primary Care Development Strategies Program*, unpublished report to The Robert Wood Johnson Foundation, 1999.

4. J. Alper, "Coming Home: Affordable Assisted Living for the Rural Elderly," *To Improve Health and Health Care 2000: The Robert Wood Johnson Foundation Anthology* (San Francisco: Jossey-Bass, 1999).

5. However, federal law requires banks to make credit available in communities where they have branches; they should not be allowed to abdicate this responsibility.

Table 10.1. Program-Related Investments of The Robert Wood Johnson Foundation.

Institution	Location	Purpose	Year Awarded	Amount
United Student Aid Funds, Inc.	Indianapolis, Indiana	Loan guarantee for medical, dental, and osteopathic students	1982	$3,000,000
On Lok Senior Health Services	San Francisco, California	Reserves support for prepaid services to health-impaired elderly	1984	$300,000
Metropolitan Jewish Geriatric Center	Brooklyn, New York	Planning, start-up, and implementation of a social HMO	1984	$300,000
New Milestones Foundation, Inc.	Austin, Texas	Housing component of the Program on Chronic Mental Illness	1988	$1,000,000
Neighborhood Properties, Inc.	Toledo, Ohio	Housing component of the Program on Chronic Mental Illness	1988	$1,000,000
Excel Development Company, Inc.	Cincinnati, Ohio	Housing component of the Program on Chronic Mental Illness	1988	$1,000,000
Community Housing Development Corp.	Charlotte, North Carolina	Housing component of the Program on Chronic Mental Illness	1988	$1,000,000
Mental Health Housing Corp. of Denver	Denver, Colorado	Housing component of the Program on Chronic Mental Illness	1988	$1,000,000
Community Housing Associates, Inc.	Baltimore, Maryland	Housing component of the Program on Chronic Mental Illness	1988	$1,001,212
Community Health Center Capital Corp.	Washington, District of Columbia	Loan guarantee for the improvement of community health centers	1989	$5,000,000

Table 10.1. Program-Related Investments of The Robert Wood Johnson Foundation, *continued*.

Institution	Location	Purpose	Year Awarded	Amount
Community Housing Network, Inc.	Columbus, Ohio	Housing component of the Program on Chronic Mental Illness	1989	$1,245,865
Our Community Hospital, Inc.	Scotland Neck, North Carolina	Construction of primary care facility	1990	$500,000
Steadfast Housing Development Corp.	Honolulu, Hawaii	Housing component of the Program on Chronic Mental Illness	1990	$1,000,000
AIDS Housing of Washington	Seattle, Washington	Model skilled nursing and adult daycare facility for persons with AIDS	1990	$1,500,000
Nevada Rural Hospital Project Foundation, Inc.	Reno, Nevada	Capitalization of a loan pool for rural hospitals	1991	$500,000
Rural Wisconsin Health Corp.	Sauk City, Wisconsin	Capitalization of a loan pool for rural hospitals	1991	$500,000
1260 Housing Development Corp.	Philadelphia, Pennsylvania	Housing component of the Program on Chronic Mental Illness	1991	$1,000,000
South Carolina Hospital Research & Education Foundation	West Columbia, South Carolina	Loan pool for conversion of M.D. practices to rural health clinics	1991	$500,000
West Alabama Health Services, Inc.	Eutaw, Alabama	Loan component of the Hospital-Based Rural Health Care Program	1991	$500,000
Community Health Facilities Fund, Inc.	Bethesda, Maryland	Loan program for agencies serving people with chronic health conditions	1991	$5,500,000
Community Health Facilities Fund, Inc.	Bethesda, Maryland	Loan program for agencies serving people with chronic health conditions	1995	$2,780,000

Table 10.1. Program-Related Investments of The Robert Wood Johnson Foundation, *continued*.

Institution	Location	Purpose	Year Awarded	Amount
New Brunswick Affiliated Hospitals, Inc.	New Brunswick, New Jersey	Construction financing completion for the Cancer Institute of New Jersey	1995	$1,000,000
Virginia Health Care Foundation	Richmond, Virginia	Loan program for health manpower retention and expansion for the Practice Sights program	1995	$700,000
Nebraska Economic Development Corp.	Lincoln, Nebraska	Loan program for health manpower retention and expansion for the Practice Sights program	1997	$1,500,000
Idaho Health Facilities Authority	Boise, Idaho	Loan program for health manpower retention and expansion for the Practice Sights program	1997	$700,000
The Minneapolis Foundation	Minneapolis, Minnesota	Loan program for health manpower retention and expansion for the Practice Sights program	1997	$1,000,000
			Total Amount	$35,027,077

~~~ Tending Our Backyard: The Robert Wood Johnson Foundation's Grantmaking in New Jersey

Pamela S. Dickson

Editors' Introduction

In sports, playing on home turf usually provides an advantage. For national philanthropies, the opposite is true: grantmaking on home turf presents a distinct disadvantage. Potential grantees in a home town or state often have very high expectations, because the distinctions between a local philanthropy and one with a national vision are difficult to understand. The Foundation's staff members, many of whom are active volunteers in local charitable organizations, can have conflicts of interest. And if an initiative close to home does not go well, relationships with neighbors can easily sour.

In this chapter, Pamela Dickson, a senior program officer at the Foundation, who oversees a number of the Foundation's New Jersey grants, tells the story of The Robert Wood Johnson Foundation's experience with grantmaking in New Jersey. Dickson has a unique vantage point; before joining the Foundation's staff in 1997, she was assistant commissioner of health for the State of New Jersey and a grantee.

Dickson reports on how the Foundation has tried to maintain the legacy of its founder, how it supports worthy local organizations that may not share The Robert Wood Johnson Foundation's priorities or may not be competitive in responding to its Calls for Proposals for national programs, and how the Foundation has tried to deal with the unique challenges of local grantmaking.

This chapter should be of interest to local readers and those interested in the Foundation's grantmaking generally. The issues that it raises go far beyond New Jersey. They are relevant to other foundations with national or state missions that want to be active in their local communities.

In 1972, The Robert Wood Johnson Foundation became a philanthropy with a national mission to improve the health and health care of all Americans. It was not, however, the birth of the foundation bearing the name of Robert Wood Johnson. The chairman and chief executive officer of Johnson & Johnson created his foundation in 1936 as a vehicle for his philanthropic endeavors in the New Brunswick area, where the company's headquarters were located.

While The Robert Wood Johnson Foundation has functioned on a national scale for 30 years, in this time it also has continued funding programs and people in the New Brunswick area and throughout New Jersey. It does so in part to honor the legacy of its founder, and in part to recognize the special responsibilities to the communities and the state in which it is located.

Every national foundation, and many foundations with a statewide focus, must balance local grantmaking with broader aims. This balancing act raises, at the outset, the question of how much should be spent locally. Other questions follow logically: what criteria should be used in deciding whom and what to fund? how closely should a foundation's overall goals guide local grantmaking? who should make local funding decisions? how can the staff effectively manage local pressures?

— The Early Years

Robert Wood Johnson (1893–1968), the son and nephew of the co-founders of the medical products giant Johnson & Johnson, grew up in an era when wealthy individuals were expected to give back a certain portion of their wealth to the community, most typically in the form of charitable assistance to the needy. Johnson began his career as a factory worker for the company at the age of 18 and spent his entire professional life with Johnson & Johnson. He became the president in 1932 and chairman of the board in 1938. While Johnson was noted at an early age for his generosity and loyalty to his home town of New Brunswick, the institutional vehicle for his gift giving was the Johnson New Brunswick Foundation, which he created in 1936 with a donation of 12,000 shares of Johnson & Johnson stock and 130 acres of land along the Raritan River in New Brunswick. The

Johnson New Brunswick Foundation was guided by a small board composed of local businessmen (inlcuding Johnson & Johnson executives), but decision-making appears to have remained squarely in Johnson's hands.[1]

The first award made by the Johnson New Brunswick Foundation was the deeding of 130 acres to the township of New Brunswick for a public park, later to be named Johnson Park. More typically, the Foundation's earliest grants were made to those down on their luck. Gifts ranged from food and clothing for poor families, to fixing an orphan boy's teeth before he departed for Boy's Town in Nebraska, to a down payment on a house for a highly regarded black policeman with a wife and eight children.

Two early grantees of the Johnson New Brunswick Foundation that remain connected to The Robert Wood Johnson Foundation to this day are Cenacle House and the Salvation Army. The residence that eventually became the retreat for the nuns of the Society of Our Lady of the Cenacle was originally the Johnson summer home, on a hilltop overlooking the Raritan River and New Brunswick. The Johnson Foundation donated the house and the grounds to the two daughters of James McGarry when they joined this order. McGarry had been a Johnson & Johnson mill superintendent who had befriended and taught Johnson the ropes in his first days with the company.

Brigadier General Henry Dries, who ran the operation of the Salvation Army in New Brunswick, recalled his first "grant proposal" by saying, "I first sought his [Johnson's] help to purchase the Hebrew Ladies' Aid Society building to house transients when they traveled between New York and Philadelphia. They were homeless, but we didn't call them that then. They were 'transients' and often alcoholics. Mr. Johnson didn't like the term 'alcoholic,' and he referred to them as 'men with drinking problems.'"[2] Despite the wide range of charitable endeavors funded by the Johnson New Brunswick Foundation, the most identifiable theme was support for the health care delivery system. Johnson cultivated an early and abiding involvement with hospital operations. He devoted funds and offered advice to the two general hospitals in New Brunswick: Middlesex General Hospital (now the Robert Wood Johnson University Hospital), where he chaired the executive committee for six years, and St. Peter's Hospital (now St. Peter's University Hospital). The Johnson New Brunswick

Foundation supported the health care professions as well, making loans so that young men from New Brunswick could go to medical school, and sponsoring programs to elevate the professional status of nurses.

In 1952, the foundation was renamed The Robert Wood Johnson Foundation. Although this name change removed the reference to New Brunswick, the foundation continued to operate locally throughout Johnson's lifetime. Johnson continued to make regular contributions of Johnson & Johnson common stock. When he died, in 1968, the Foundation held 569,130 shares, with a value of $60,000,000.

⸻ Outgrowing New Brunswick

Johnson left the bulk of his estate, consisting of Johnson & Johnson stock then valued at $300 million, to the Foundation. By the time probate was concluded, in 1971, the value of the shares had increased fourfold, to $1.2 billion.

Johnson did not stipulate a focus for these funds other than a general hope that they would benefit mankind. There are no minutes that reflect the trustees' decision to promote the betterment of the health of the American people, but it seems an obvious choice, in the light of Johnson's business and personal interests over his lifetime. Given the size of the assets, the trustees decided that the Foundation should assume a national presence.

The Foundation's first chairman was Gustav Lienhard, who was at the time president of Johnson & Johnson. Lienhard, who served as the Foundation's chairman and CEO until 1986, exerted great influence over the Foundation's early development, broadening its reach well beyond New Brunswick and New Jersey. He also stressed a businesslike attitude toward grantmaking, indicating a preference for sustainability and replicability in projects funded by the Foundation. Lienhard and the new board also underscored the Foundation's focus on health by selecting as its first president Dr. David E. Rogers, the dean of the Johns Hopkins University School of Medicine. Rogers selected a program staff with national expertise in various health policy fields and developed a series of demonstration projects with sites throughout the nation.

In the 1972 *Annual Report*, Rogers laid out a 17-page analysis of health care opportunities and strategies, and identified three national program strategies for the Foundation:

- Improving access to medical care for underserved Americans
- Improving the quality of health and medical care
- Developing mechanisms for objective analysis of public policies in health

The staff was asked to develop program priorities that would achieve these goals, and the Foundation developed a new model of grantmaking for its national programs—one that identified, in advance, a program's goals and criteria for grantee selection. This was very different from the approach used by most national foundations at the time, which tended to respond to unsolicited proposals for funds.

Even as this national perspective was being developed, local institutions saw the increase in the Foundation's assets as an opportunity to receive even more support than in the past. Recalling Johnson's generosity and anticipating the Foundation's help in purchasing land, new equipment, and other capital expansions, New Brunswick hospitals and other health care institutions made plans for capital improvements.

In the early days, the biggest challenge facing the young Foundation was meeting the new 7 percent payout required by the Tax Reform Act of 1969 (later reduced to 5 percent). As a result of the large payout requirement, little competition for resources emerged initally. Although tensions about whether to allocate funds locally or nationally surfaced occasionally in meetings of the board of trustees throughout the 1970s and 1980s, the board did not appear to have adopted a formal position on the matter. Requests for local funding were presented, reviewed, and funded on an informal basis.

The necessity of dealing with this issue came to a head, however, in the late 1980s, when the staff decided to take another look at what seemed like a continuous list of requests from Middlesex General Hospital. Once the small project budgets were aggregated, the total came to $10 million. Given the level of funding requested, the board decided to develop a more formal policy and process to guide its central New Jersey giving. In 1990, the board adopted a resolution that central New Jersey grants "remain at 3 percent of the Foundation's total annual grantmaking, as calculated on a five-year average." The 3 percent figure was adopted as a continuation of past trends, and was seen as more of a target than a cap. However, the Foundation's giving to local charities that reflected Robert Wood Johnson's legacy from the 1930s were considered above and beyond the 3 percent target.

⎯ The Foundation's New Jersey Funding

Decisions about how much to allocate to local versus national programs, for what purposes, and how to do so reflect a complicated history and an interplay of dynamic forces ranging from the founders' wishes to the degree of specificity with which the Foundation defines its goals and the successes or failures of past grantmaking. The Robert Wood Johnson Foundation's current New Jersey funding can be sorted into four different categories:

- *Legacy Grants* are, in general, charitable donations to organizations in the New Brunswick area that were supported by, or similar to those supported by, Johnson before The Robert Wood Johnson Foundation adopted a national perspective.

- *Out-of-Program Grants* are made to New Jersey organizations, predominantly in the New Brunswick area, for programs that are generally consistent with the Foundation's goals but do not necessarily fall within its priorities.

- *In-Program Grants* are expected to meet the Foundation's overall goals and more specific programming priorities. These grants are earmarked for New Jersey organizations that compete only with other New Jersey applicants.

- *National Program Grants* are made to New Jersey applicants that successfully compete with other applicants throughout the nation.

Legacy Grants

Giving to New Brunswick charities, a valued tradition for the Foundation's board, is seen as a way of honoring the Foundation's founder. Programs funded as legacy grants do not have to fall within the Foundation's mandate, nor do they go through a competitive selection process. In this regard, they are akin to the charitable donations of a community foundation. Legacy grants fund the same New Brunswick charities that were supported by Robert Wood Johnson in his early days as a philanthropist, as well as other local groups carrying out similar charitable endeavors. The Salvation Army, the Society of St. Vincent de Paul, Cenacle Retreat House, the Central New Jersey United Way of Central New Jersey, the Plainsboro Rescue Squad and Plainsboro Volunteer Fire Company No. 1 (the Foundation's headquarters are in Plainsboro Township), and Kiddie Keep Well Camp (a summer camp available to children with severe illness or disabilities) are among the organizations that The Robert Wood Johnson Foundation has supported for many years.

New Brunswick went through a very difficult economic period in the 1970s; it rebounded in the 1990s, and has become a thriving city. Part of the recovery can be credited to Johnson & Johnson's decision to maintain its headquarters in the city, and part can also be given to the ongoing support of The Robert Wood Johnson Foundation. The Foundation has given core support to two municipal organizations: New Brunswick Tomorrow, a network of human service agencies, and the New Brunswick Development Corporation, charged with rebuilding the downtown area.

For the most part, these grantees are sustained with annual increases adjusted for the cost of living. Funding in this category throughout the 1990s was approximately $14 million.

⟡

Table 11.1.   Selected Legacy Grants.

Grantee	Year Funded	2000 Funding
Cenacle Retreat House	1949	$72,000
Salvation Army	1972	$250,000
Kiddie Keep Well Camp	1975	$322,000
New Brunswick Development Corporation Corporation	1981 1981	$300,000 $300,000
New Brunswick Tomorrow	1977	$350,000
United Way of Central Jersey	1976	$550,000
Society of St. Vincent de Paul	1972	$132,000

Out-of-Program Grants

Under the 1990 board resolution, out-of-program grants are targeted at 3 percent of the Foundation's annual grant giving. Like legacy grants, out-of-program awards do not have to fall within the Foundation's strategic priorities. But unlike the legacy grants, which tend to be small and sustained with small increments over many years, out-of-program grants tend to be large one-time awards, even when they are made to beneficiaries that were early recipients of Johnson's largesse. Although it's not a requirement that out-of-program grants be related to health care, they tend to be so; they are typically awarded to central New Jersey health care organizations. This category of grants, together with the legacy grants, comes closest to fulfilling the Foundation's role as a good corporate neighbor. Out-of-program grants reflect a sense of pride in the state of New Jersey and an acknowledgement of its importance in the lives of Robert Wood Johnson, Johnson & Johnson, and most of the early trustees.

Many of the Foundation's out-of-program grants have gone to increase the capacity of New Jersey's health care institutions, so that the state's residents could have access to first-rate medical facilities without having to go to New York City or Philadelphia. In its earlier days, the Foundation focused on strengthening the University of Medicine and Dentistry of New Jersey, which had its headquarters in Newark and teaching sites in New Brunswick and Camden, and

Table 11.2. Selected Out-of-Program Grants.

Grantee	Year Funded	Amount
New Jersey Cardiovascular Institute	2001	$10,000,000
Child Health Institute of New Jersey	1998	$5,500,000
	2001	$10,000,000
Cancer Institute of New Jersey	1999	$6,000,000
	2001	$10,000,000
Center for State Health Policy at Rutgers	1998	$11,000,000

supporting other health care providers in Middlesex County, like the Robert Wood Johnson, Jr., Rehabilitation Institute. More recently, the Foundation made major capital gifts to help establish the New Jersey Cancer Center, the New Jersey Cardiovascular Institute, and a new Child Health Institute, all of which are in New Brunswick.

Another out-of-program grant established the Center for State Health Policy at Rutgers University in 1999. The Center aims at serving the state in two ways. First, it focuses Rutgers' academic resources on health policy development, giving it the potential to become a nationally recognized institution in this field. Second, it provides advice—based on the university's health-related expertise across a range of disciplines—to the state government. To increase the usefulness of this function, the Center brings together teams of researchers and subject-matter specialists able to respond quickly to requests from state health care decision makers for background information, research findings, and policy analyses. During the 1990s, $64 million was approved for projects in this category.

In-Program Grants

In-Program Grants occupy a middle ground between the Foundation's legacy and out-of-program grants—with their comparatively informal review process—and its national program grants—with their rigorous selection process. In-program grants are made only to New Jersey organizations for activities that fall within the priorities of the Foundation.

The rationale for creating a middle ground that gives preferential treatment to home state applicants is threefold. First, if good ideas are being put into practice elsewhere, then the Foundation ought to be sure that New Jersey also benefits. Second, such grants encourage the testing of innovative ideas in the Foundation's home state. Third, they help build health and health care expertise in New Jersey.

As the young Robert Wood Johnson Foundation began to roll out its large national programs in the 1970s, a highly competitive and rigorous process developed in which a large number of applicants would submit proposals in response to a Call for Proposals. Often, New Jersey applicants were not successful in securing grants. However, the Foundation liked the idea of including a New Jersey site when it made awards in its nationwide programs, and, as a result, it became common practice to add a New Jersey site when the successful applicant pool did not include a New Jersey organization. Eventually, the Foundation chose another route that would give preference to organizations within its home state: the New Jersey Health Initiatives.

The initial proposal to establish the New Jersey Health Initiatives, submitted to the board of trustees in December of 1986, requested the authorization of funds for "a visible effort providing seed-money grants for unusual health care innovations" within the state. It expressed the hope that the program would create an impetus for New Jersey institutions to move more rapidly in health and health care, and would provide a mechanism for assessing many of the proposals the Foundation routinely received from institutions around the state.

Under the New Jersey Health Initiatives, organizations across the state have an opportunity to respond to Calls for Proposals, issued once or twice a year, that solicit innovative community-based projects addressing one or more of the Foundation's goal areas—currently, increasing access to care, improving prevention and treatment

---

✦

Table 11.3.   Selected In-Program New Jersey Grants.

Grantee	Year Funded	Amount
Alliance of Community Health Plans —Tobacco control in physician networks	2000	$475,000
Foundation at New Jersey Institute of Technology —Videotape for parents of disabled children	2000	$181,000
New Jersey Health Policy Forums	2000	$649,000
Caucus Education Corporation —Health care series on public television	1999	$151,000
New Jersey Minority Health Summit	1999	$50,000

of chronic illness, promoting healthy communities and lifestyles, and reducing the harm caused by substance abuse. The Foundation will fund grants up to $500,000 over a three-year period.

As it often does with national programs, The Robert Wood Johnson Foundation designated an outside organization to administer the New Jersey Health Initiatives. Not only does this reduce the Foundation's administrative burden and tap into expertise beyond the Foundation's walls, but it also reduces the pressure on the staff from local applicants.

The first program office, beginning in January of 1987, was the Health Corporation of the Archdiocese of Newark. In the mid-1990s, the program office shifted to the Health Research and Educational Trust of New Jersey in Princeton. In 2001, the program home changed once again to the Institute for Health, Health Care Policy and Aging Research at Rutgers University. In each of its various homes, the New Jersey Health Initiatives staff manages the process in conjunction with an outside review committee. This process includes proposal review, selection of grantees, and grant administration. With the help of the advisory committee, the staff recommends to the Foundation the best candidates out of each pool for funding.

Some New Jersey Health Initiatives projects have been noteworthy. The Monmouth Medical Center, for example, organized interdisciplinary teams of medical and social service professionals to coordinate services for dying patients. The project was favorably received by patients' families, and the hospital staff was so enthusiastic that the hospital arranged relief time for staff members who wanted to participate. It became a model that the Foundation used as it was developing strategies to improve palliative care for dying patients. Another example is the New Jersey SEED Project, which supported the development of ethics training to facilitate dispute resolution in nursing homes. Although the state of New Jersey funds regional long-term-care ethics committees that offer general guidance, their resources are insufficient to provide guidance on the specific issues that arise in the care of individuals in nursing homes. The grant enabled in-house training to be made available to the staffs of many New Jersey long-term care facilities.

In addition to the New Jersey Health Initiatives, the Foundation also funds unsolicited proposals that have the potential for local impact. An example is the Capitol Policy Forums project. Early in the

1990s, the League of Women Voters of New Jersey requested the Foundation's financial support in an effort to promote a more civil discourse on important health policy issues in New Jersey. In response, the Foundation agreed to fund a series of quarterly forums on key health issues, sponsored by the League of Women Voters of New Jersey and attended by state public policymakers and stakeholders. The Foundation continues to support these forums, now sponsored by the Forums Institute for Public Policy, and has financed similar efforts in other states.

The Foundation has also undertaken several initiatives with the New Jersey state government. In the 1980s, it contributed to the state's establishment of seven hospital consortia to transfer pregnant women with potentially high-risk deliveries to hospitals best prepared to care for endangered newborns. The funding for these consortiums has been picked up by member hospitals, and they remain in operation today.

In response to a request from the state government, the Foundation funded, between 1996 and 2000, an innovative way to monitor quality of care in nursing homes. The traditional approach involved facility inspections based largely on physical plant standards and staffing levels. However, these criteria did not measure actual resident outcomes. In the mid-1990s, the federal Health Care Financing Administration was beginning the process of creating quality-of-care indicators for nursing home residents that could be reported in an electronic format. New Jersey proposed that the new federal electronic database also be used by its state inspectors—not in a punitive way but to help nursing homes set quality-of-care goals for themselves.

The Foundation has also funded capacity-building projects in the state government. Len Fishman, Commissioner of Health from 1993 through 1998, relates that he was thrilled with the flexibility of a $50,000 award from the Foundation to be used on a health policy issue of his choosing. Later in his term, a Foundation grant enabled the Department of Health and two other state agencies to carry out a comprehensive planning process based on consolidating into a single agency all of the state's services to the elderly. That funding "brought many more people to the table than would otherwise have been possible," observed Fishman.

Over the decade of the 1990s, the Foundation made 286 in-program New Jersey grants totaling $86 million.

National Program Grants

New Jersey organizations, like those from any other state, can respond to Calls for Proposals and seek funds for national programs in areas identified as priorities by The Robert Wood Johnson Foundation. New Jersey applicants receive no special advantages in these competitions, and, like applicants from any state, face tough odds in them. There are, however, some outstanding examples of New Jersey grantees having competed successfully. For example, the New Jersey Breathes project, run by the New Jersey Medical Society, was one of the original nine sites in the SmokeLess States program. New Jersey Breathes and its partners in the state engaged in public education about the harmful impact of cigarette smoking among young people. The issue received widespread attention, and, in 1997, the state cigarette tax was increased.

—— Conclusion

As currently structured, the Foundation's New Jersey grantmaking maintains certain of its central values, principally by honoring its founder, serving as a corporate good neighbor, standing behind grantees' work rather than seeking the spotlight, and encouraging innovative ideas for improving health and health care in its home state. The Foundation's approach to grantmaking in New Jersey has significantly different emphases than its national approach. While in its national programs the Foundation issues Calls for Proposals that have the potential to shape policies, to build new fields, and to demonstrate innovative ideas that others might pick up, its approach in New Jersey is to respond to local initiatives and, to a great extent, to fund community-based programs. This approach offers a more receptive environment for a wide range of proposals, especially those that do not fall within the Foundation's national goals. This approach has both benefits and costs. These can be seen by examining four issues that arise from the Foundation's New Jersey grantmaking: What is an appropriate amount for a national foundation to give for programs in its own backyard? What are appropriate program priorities? What is an appropriate mechanism for making funding decisions? How visible should a national foundation be locally?

Funding level

The first issue involves deciding how much of its funds a national foundation such as Robert Wood Johnson should devote to its own backyard. In 1990, the Foundation determined that, given past expenditures, a 3 percent level for out-of-program grants would be appropriate. Using historical spending patterns as a yardstick may be a rational way to determine current spending levels, but it has the potential drawback of freezing local grantmaking at a level based only on history. However, the Foundation built in flexibility: The 3 percent is merely a target—a level that it should try to reach. Second, the 3 percent target applies only to out-of-program grants; in-program grants, including the New Jersey Health Initiatives, legacy grants, and, of course, grants to New Jersey applicants in national competitions are above and beyond the 3 percent. The exclusion of legacy grants in the 3 percent target is understandable, since the number of legacy grantees is finite, predetermined, and continuing, whereas the demand for out-of program grants to facilities and institutions is considerably less predictable. By excluding in-program grants from the 3 percent set-aside, these projects, in effect, compete for funds with the Foundation's national grantmaking portfolio.

Program Priorities

The second issue concerns the activities that fall within the guidelines for local grantmaking. The Foundation has program priorities in New Jersey different from those it has in other states. In New Jersey, the Foundation acts, for the most part, as a traditional community foundation, funding local charitable endeavors and using guidelines quite different from those it uses nationally. Its emphasis on charitable giving through the legacy and out-of-program mechanisms—whether or not they involve health—is markedly different from the Foundation's program priorities elsewhere. Even the New Jersey Health Initiatives, in which projects must fit within the Foundation's priorities, looks for community-based service activities and excludes grants for policy and research, which are a primary tool in many national programs.

Moreover, like community foundations that usually react to proposals that come over the transom, the Foundation makes grants that respond to requests coming from community organizations in New Jersey; this contrasts with its more structured and activist approach to national programs. Responding to the needs defined by local organizations is part of the definition of being a good corporate neighbor.

Some critics have commented that the approach the Foundation has adopted in New Jersey may deprive it of the opportunity to play a more decisive role in the state. In response to the challenge of making a greater impact in New Jersey, the board approved an expanded scope for the New Jersey Health Initiatives in July, 2001, adding three new elements: a community leadership program, capacity-building for community organizations, and a strategic Call for Proposals in which each cycle will target a particular health or health care issue.

Mechanisms for Decision-Making

A third issue is how to make decisions about what organizations and projects to fund. The Foundation's program staff is essentially removed from most New Jersey program development and decision-making. Legacy and out-of-program grants do not go through the normal staff proposal review process; review and decisions are basically made by committees of the board of trustees. Decision-making on New Jersey Health Initiatives grants is in the hands of an external program office, although members of the Foundation's program staff with relevant experience may be asked to comment on specific proposals.

The separation of the Foundation's program staff from grantmaking in New Jersey has its pros and cons. It has the benefit of shielding the staff from involvement in projects that may have been submitted by friends or neighbors. Additionally, the use of an expert advisory committee and a competitive review process for in-program grants funded under the New Jersey Health Initiatives maintains the credibility of the grantmaking process. However, the advantages brought by distancing the staff from local projects comes at a price: the Foundation loses the opportunity to apply its strategic and time-tested grantmaking process in New Jersey, and the staff is less able to share insights gained from its national programs with local audiences.

The Foundation's Visibility

Mark Murphy, executive director of the Fund for New Jersey, is not shy about expressing his admiration for The Robert Wood Johnson Foundation. However, he considers the Foundation's preference for remaining in the background among its less effective characteristics. He points out that the Foundation has learned much from projects all over the country that should inform the Foundation's potential to effect positive change in New Jersey. "The Robert Wood Johnson Foundation is uniquely positioned to provide expertise and resources to bring people together and make things happen," Murphy said. "The process that has protected the Foundation from the stickiness of engagement has also protected it from some of the potential achievements of engagement."

The Foundation's preference for low visibility is not unique to New Jersey. Indeed, it goes back to its first board chairman, Gustav Lienhard, and was reaffirmed as recently as 1999 with the board's adoption of a set of core values, including this: "We speak through our grantees and do not seek a high institutional profile." Without abandoning this core value, however, the Foundation could use the power of its New Jersey funding more strategically. Pauline Seitz, director of the New Jersey Health Initiatives through the end of 2000, took steps in this direction by using the Initiative's quasi-community foundation status to become active in the Council of New Jersey Grantmakers. As vice-president, she stimulated discussion about how New Jersey philanthropies could pool their assets for the good of the state.

How could the Foundation strengthen the impact of its New Jersey funding without losing the benefits of the approach that has evolved over the years? One way would be to adopt a strategic approach that would establish New Jersey as a discrete goal area, subject to the same incentives, constraints, and performance assessment that are applied to the national grantmaking processes. Two-way communications that would facilitate the sharing of experiences between New Jersey grantees and national program grantees could be built into the approach, and a budget process could be developed that would identify an appropriate level of resources needed to reach the goals.

A second approach would be to develop in selected localities in New Jersey what is referred to as a "place-based" type of grantmaking. Rather than taking one model and seeking to replicate it in many different sites, the place-based site approach takes many different types of interventions and implements them in a single place. The multiple interventions might yield synergies where the whole is greater than the sum of its parts. For several years, the Foundation has discussed applying this approach to children's health in a city in New Jersey. In

July, 2001, the board approved the Children's Futures program, which will focus exclusively on Trenton and bring to bear all that the Foundation has learned about improving the health of children between the ages of 0 and 3. This initiative might be risky because of the potential involvement of the Foundation in local affairs, but it could make a genuine and lasting contribution to the Foundation's home state.[3]

Notes

1. The source for material about the life of Robert Wood Johnson is Lawrence Foster, *Robert Wood Johnson: The Gentleman Rebel* (State College, Pennsylvania: Lillian Press, 1999).
2. Ibid, p. 371.
3. The author would like to thank the following people for their insights and contributions toward this chapter: Len Fishman, Lawrence G. Foster, Ruby Hearn, Robert G. Hughes Frank Karel, Terrance Keenan, Mark Murphy, Mary Quinn, Pauline Seitz, and Warren Wood.

⌁ The Editors

Stephen L. Isaacs, J.D., is the president of Health Policy Associates in San Francisco. A former professor of public health at Columbia University and founding director of its Development Law and Policy Program, he has written extensively for professional and popular audiences. His book *The Consumer's Legal Guide to Today's Health Care* was reviewed as "the single best guide to the health care system in print today;" his articles have been widely syndicated and have appeared in law reviews and health policy journals. He also provides technical assistance internationally on health law, civil society, and social policy. A graduate of Brown University and Columbia Law School, Mr. Isaacs served as vice president of International Planned Parenthood's Latin American division, practiced health law, and spent four years in Thailand as a program officer for the U.S. Agency for International Development.

James R. Knickman, Ph.D., is vice president for research and evaluation at The Robert Wood Johnson Foundation. He oversees a range of grants and national programs supporting research and policy analysis to better understand forces that can improve health status and the delivery of health care. In addition, he is in charge of developing formal evaluations of national programs supported by the Foundation. He has also played a leadership role in developing grant-making strategy in the areas of chronic illness, long-term care, and population health during his nine years at the Foundation. During the 1999–2000 academic year, he held a Regents' Lectureship at the University of California, Berkeley. Previously, Dr. Knickman was on the faculty of the Robert F. Wagner Graduate School of Public Service at New York University. Currently, he is vice-chair of the board of trustees of Robert Wood Johnson University Hospital in New Brunswick. He completed his undergraduate work at Fordham University and received his doctorate in public policy analysis from the University of Pennsylvania.

—— The Contributors

Joseph Alper has been a science and health care writer for 21 years. During that time, he has served as a contributing correspondent for *Science,* and as a contributing editor of *Nature Biotechnology* and *Self* magazines. He has also written for a variety of publications, including *The Atlantic Monthly, Harper's, The New York Times, The Washington Post,* and *Health Magazine,* and has written numerous policy documents for the National Institutes of Health and the National Academy of Sciences. Alper has won several national writing awards, including the American Chemical Society's Grady/Stack Award for career achievements in science writing and two national writing awards from the American Psychological Association. Alper has also taught journalism and writing at the University of Wisconsin at Madison, Johns Hopkins University, the University of Minnesota, and Colorado State University. He graduated from the University of Illinois at Urbana, and received Master's of Science degrees in both Biochemistry and Agricultural Journalism from the University of Wisconsin at Madison.

A. E. (Ted) Benjamin, Ph.D., is professor and chair in the Department of Social Welfare, School of Public Policy and Social Research at the University of California, Los Angeles. His interests include long-term services for people with chronic conditions, particularly comparative access and quality issues. He has done research on various populations with chronic health conditions in order to better understand commonalities and differences and their impact on public policy. This research has involved the elderly, younger adults with chronic condition, people with HIV disease, and children with special health needs. His most recent research has addressed consumer direction in home care with support from the U.S. Department of Health and Human Services and The Robert Wood Johnson Foundation. He has written numerous papers on home and community-based services and is co-editor (with Bob Newcomer) of *Indicators of Chronic Health Conditions,* published in 1997 by Johns Hopkins University Press. He received a doctorate in political science and social work from the University of Michigan in 1977.

Paul Brodeur was a staff writer at *The New Yorker* for nearly forty years. During that time, he alerted the nation to the public health hazard posed by asbestos, to the depletion of the ozone layer by chlorofluorocarbons, and to the harmful effects of microwave radiation and power-frequency electromagnetic fields. His work has been acknowledged with a National Magazine Award and the Journalism Award of the American Association for the Advancement of Science. The United Nations Environment Program has named him to its Global 500 Roll of Honour for outstanding environmental achievements.

Ethan Bronner was named education editor at *The New York Times* in 1999. He came to *The New York Times* in September 1997 as a national correspondent and reported on trends in higher education and grades K through 12. From 1985 until 1997, Mr. Bronner was with *The Boston Globe*, where he served as Middle East correspondent, based in Jerusalem, and a Supreme Court and legal affairs correspondent in Washington, D.C. He began his journalistic career at Reuters in 1980 and reported from London, Madrid, Brussels, and Jerusalem. Mr. Bronner is the author of *Battle for Justice: How the Bork Nomination Shook America*, which was chosen by the New York Public Library as one of the 25 best books of 1989. Mr. Bronner received a B.A. in Letters from Wesleyan University and an M.S. from Columbia University's School of Journalism.

Susan Dentzer is the on-air health correspondent for *The NewsHour* with Jim Lehrer on PBS, where she leads a unit devoted to coverage of a wide range of health and medical topics. The unit is a partnership between *The NewsHour* and the Henry J. Kaiser Family Foundation. Many of Dentzer's pieces focus on policy issues, such as Social Security and Medicare reform, the uninsured and growing needs for long-term care. In 2000, Dentzer was awarded the Robinson Electronic Media Award by the American Psychiatric Association for her report on schizophrenia. Both a print and a television journalist, Dentzer was formerly chief economics correspondent and economics columnist for *U.S. News & World Report* and a senior writer at *Newsweek*. A graduate of Dartmouth College and a former Nieman Fellow at Harvard University, Dentzer is currently chair of the Dartmouth Board of Trustees.

Pamela S. Dickson is a senior program officer at The Robert Wood Johnson Foundation. Her program activities at the Foundation focus on increasing access to care for all Americans, with a particular emphasis on reducing racial and ethnic disparities in access to care; as well as contributions to the Foundation's New Jersey funding portfolio. Before joining the Foundation, Ms. Dickson held several senior positions at the New Jersey Department of Health, including assistant commissioner from 1988 through 1994 and a subsequent term as director of health care reform initiatives. Ms. Dickson has held positions as a member of the Board of Directors of the National Association of Health Data Organizations and of the Access for the Uninsured Steering Committee of the National Academy for State Health Policy. She holds an M.B.A. in Health Care Administration from the Wharton School of Business.

Digby Diehl is a writer, a literary collaborator, and a television, print, and internet journalist. Recently honored with the Jack Smith Award from the Friends of the Pasadena Public Library, his book credits include *Angel on My Shoulder*, the autobiography of singer Natalie Cole; *The Million Dollar Mermaid*, the autobiography of MGM star Esther Williams; *Tales from the Crypt*, the history of the popular comic book, movie, and television series; and *A Spy for All Seasons*, the autobiography of former CIA officer Duane Clarridge. For eleven years, Diehl was the literary correspondent for ABC-TV's *Good Morning America*, and was recently the book editor for the *Home Page* show on MSNBC. He continues to appear regularly on the Morning News on KTLA. Previously the entertainment editor for KCBS television in Los Angeles, he was a writer for the Emmys and for the soap opera *Santa Barbara*, book editor of the *Los Angeles Herald Examiner*, editor-in-chief of art book publishers Harry N. Abrams, Inc., and the founding book editor of *The Los Angeles Times Book Review*. Diehl holds an M.A. in Theatre from UCLA and a B.A. in American Studies from Rutgers University, where he was a Henry Rutgers Scholar.

Richard S. Frank is a freelance writer and editor and is currently an adjunct professor at Boston University's Washington Journalism Center. From 1976 to 1997, he was the editor of *National Journal*, the Washington-based weekly on national politics and federal policy. During his tenure, the magazine won two National Magazine Awards and its reporters won numerous national awards for public affairs reporting. His earlier journalistic experience included stints as a local government reporter for the *Bergen Record* in New Jersey, as a statehouse and City Hall reporter for the *Baltimore Evening Sun,* as state legislative correspondent and public transportation reporter and Washington correspondent for the *Philadelphia Bulletin,* and as international economics and trade reporter, associate editor, and managing editor at *National Journal.* He interrupted his journalistic career for almost two years to serve as chief administrative assistant to the Mayor of Baltimore. He has a bachelor's degree from Syracuse University in international relations and journalism and a master's from the University of Chicago in political science, and he was an Advanced International Reporting Fellow at Columbia University.

Peter Goodwin is vice president and treasurer at The Robert Wood Johnson Foundation. Before he joined the Foundation, in 1984, he was administrator at the Beth Israel Medical Center, New York. In 1991, he was promoted to vice president for financial monitoring and in 1995 promoted to treasurer. He oversees the areas of treasury, accounting, information technology, financial monitoring, and administration. He is chairman of the Board of Directors at the Sikora Center in Camden, New Jersey, a member of the Board of Directors of the Haddonfield Little League, and was a 1995 Fellow in Leadership New Jersey. He received his bachelor's degree from Boston College and his MBA in Health Care Administration and Finance from Baruch College, City University of New York.

Marco Navarro is a program officer at The Robert Wood Johnson Foundation. He is a member of the Community Health and Health and Behavior program management teams. Navarro became a program officer after five years as a financial officer for the Foundation. Before joining the Foundation, he worked for ten years managing community development programs, including the production of affordable housing projects and the growth of a community-owned credit union in the City of Newark, New Jersey. Mr. Navarro earned a master's degree in city and regional planning from Rutgers University, and has served as a public commissioner of the New Jersey Urban Enterprise Zone Authority since 1989.

Carolyn Newbergh is a Northern California writer who has covered health care trends and policy issues for more than 20 years. Her freelance work has appeared in numerous print and online publications.

As a reporter for the *Oakland Tribune*, Ms. Newbergh wrote articles on health care delivery for the poor as well as emergency room violence, AIDS, and the impact of crack cocaine on the children of addicts. Ms. Newbergh was also an investigative reporter for the *Tribune*, winning prestigious honors for a series on how consultants intentionally cover up earthquake hazards in California.

Richard C. Reynolds, M.D., is a courtesy professor of medicine at the University of Florida College of Medicine. In his previous role as executive vice president at The Robert Wood Johnson Foundation, he participated in the development and oversight of several programs in medical education. He is a former dean of The Robert Wood Johnson Medical School and a senior vice president for academic affairs at the University of Medicine and Dentistry of New Jersey. Previously, while a faculty member at the University of Florida, he helped initiate a program in general internal medicine and became the founding chairman of the Department of Community Health and Family Medicine. He has co-edited two books, *Health of a Rural County* and *On Doctoring*. Trained as an internist, he first practiced in a small city in western Maryland.

Steven A. Schroeder, M.D., is president and chief executive officer of The Robert Wood Johnson Foundation. A graduate of Stanford University and Harvard Medical School, Dr. Schroeder trained in internal medicine at the Harvard Medical Service of the Boston City Hospital, in epidemiology as a member of the Epidemic Intelligence Service of the Communicable Diseases Center, and in public health at the Harvard Center for Community Health and Medical Care. He served as an instructor in medicine at Harvard, assistant and associate professor of medicine and health care sciences at George Washington University, and associate professor and professor of medicine at the University of California, San Francisco (UCSF). At both George Washington University and UCSF he was founding medical director of a university-sponsored health maintenance organization, and at UCSF he founded its Division of General Internal Medicine. Dr. Schroeder continues to practice general internal medicine on a part-time basis at the Robert Wood Johnson Medical School. He has more than 225 publications to his credit. Dr. Schroeder has served on a number of editorial boards, including—at present—the *New England Journal of Medicine*, and is a member of the boards of the International Academic Review Committee for the Goldman School of Medicine, Ben-Gurion University of the Negev, Israel, the American Legacy Foundation, and the Harvard University Board of Overseers. He has received honorary doctorates from Rush University, Boston University, the University of Massachusetts, and Georgetown University.

Rani E. Snyder, M.P.A., is a research associate at the School of Public Policy and Social Research at the University of California, Los Angeles, and a doctoral student at the UCLA School of Public Health. Her work has focused mainly on issues affecting elderly people and the Medicare program and includes publications in *Health Affairs, Medical Care Research and Review*, and *Health Services Research*. Prior to moving to Los Angeles, she worked at two foundations that fund work in health care: the John A. Hartford Foundation and the Commonwealth Fund. She has a master's degree in public administration from New York University.

John Stone, M.D., is professor of medicine (cardiology) and associate dean at Emory University School of Medicine. A clinician and teacher, he is also a writer and poet whose work has appeared widely, from *The New York Times Magazine* to *Poetry* (Chicago). He has written four books of poetry, all from Louisiana State University Press; the most recent is *Where Water Begins* (1998). *In the Country of Hearts* is a collection of his writings about his career in cardiology. He has spoken and read from his work in 38 states and at more than 100 institutions from Yale to Stanford to Oxford University, England.

Index

Table of Contents

To Improve Health and Health Care 1997

~~~ Table of Contents

To Improve Health and Health Care 1998–1999

~~~ Table of Contents

To Improve Health and Health Care 2000

—⁓— **Table of Contents**

To Improve Health and Health Care 2001